Unapologetically
Able

Unapologetically Able by Chaeli Mycroft
ISBN: 978-0-620-92678-2   Print
ISBN: 978-0-620-92777-2   Digital

Self-published by Michaela Mycroft
Cover Design: King James Group
Editor: Paula Hepburn-Brown

(they said I'd never be able to write... haha)

For Damian
You were so excited to see this story told.
I miss you every day, partner.

CONTENTS

FOREWORD

Whatever has led to you picking up this book, opening it and reading it, welcome. I'm so happy you're here.

One thing I would like you to take with you as you make your way through my story, as you turn each page is this... I haven't written this book to be a source of inspiration. It's just my story – a collection of memories, experiences, lessons and ideas of plans for the future. I want to give you the inside track on what living with disability means, for me. I want to share the hilarity, the difficulties, the confusion, the successes and the failures. I'm not here to say I know what I'm doing or that I have any valuable advice to give. I don't see myself as an expert on anything (except maybe my own thoughts and feelings). A lot of the time I am really confused and anxious about what's happening in my life and I constantly question whether I'm doing the right thing and making the right choices. I know, though, that life is made by the small moments of bravery and our stories come from what happens after those moments.

I wrote this book to share this really complicated journey of living with my disability – the laughter, the tears, the excitement, the stress ... all of it. I haven't been on Earth for too long, but in this time I have lived, and continue to live, a crazy, full life. Writing things down and sharing stories is me trying to figure out how to make it through life relatively successfully and figuring out what that even means. I'm taking this moment to reflect on what has happened so far, and I'm looking forward to the coming decades.

Please pay attention to the mini side note thoughts and [TANGENTS] throughout these stories too, as they might give you some insight into how my mind works... I'm also a super sarcastic human, and sarcasm is one of my key communication methods, so get ready.

If you read something here that resonates with you, or you can relate and have had a similar experience, awesome. If you read something in here that you completely disagree with, cool. I want these stories to get you thinking; to start a conversation. Maybe I can change a few perspectives and maybe it will solidify a view that you have. I'm excited for all of it.

Are you ready?

Am I?

Okay, deep breath.

Let's do this.

PART 1: FINDING MY FEET

Chapter 1
This is my life

CONTEXTUALISING MY DISABILITY

To begin, I'd like to share some basic information that I feel is important for you to know so that you can have a better understanding of my life and how things have worked out. I live my life in a wheelchair, with cerebral palsy (CP) and a degenerative neuropathy (which, to be honest, we haven't really paid too much attention to, but I'll explain why in a minute). My disability is a big deal to a lot of people. It's obviously a big deal to me too, for a whole lot of reasons. It has definitely played a role in shaping my life in interesting and important ways, but it isn't the *only* thing that has shaped my life. I have a lot of other things going on – I'd love you to remember this as we go through these chapters and I take you through my life experiences (the good, the bad and the learning).

Disability can be complicated to understand and to experience, and it's okay if you're confused or don't understand all the nuances of why things are the way they are or why disabled people respond in particular ways to certain circumstances and conversations. I get it. I'm confused a lot of the time too! I often end up on both sides of the fence in discussions exactly because of this complicated nature of disability in our able-centric world. It's important to acknowledge that disability fills a space in society that is under the radar and it makes a lot of people uncomfortable. I've learnt to be comfortable in the discomfort of people who don't yet see the value disability can and does bring to our communities; who haven't realised it's an enriching experience when people embrace it with all of its intricacies. I have to believe they'll come round. I have had my disability for as long as I can remember, so you'd think a quarter of a century (plus one year) into this life I should or would have it down by now. But it's not that simple...

Living with a disability is an evolution (for me and everyone in my life). It's an experience that constantly challenges my understanding of myself, of other people, of the world around me and of my role in it. It's a journey of continuous self-discovery and I'm excited that I get to bring you along with me as I dive back into what has led to this point in my life.

I have been a wheelchair user for basically my whole life. Technically, I was three when I got my first wheelchair. The smallest chair they could get in South Africa was a 40cm adult wheelchair because the chairs for children my size weren't yet available in the country. These were also incredibly expensive and we couldn't afford one. I have never been able to walk independently, so I don't miss walking or anything. It's never been a part of my life (or as Andie from *How to Lose a Guy in 10 Days* put it: "You can't lose something you never had"), so don't feel bad. I'm cool with it. The part of me that embraces laziness and staying home to binge-watch series for a week, eating copious amounts of unhealthy but soul-serving snacks, enjoys the fact that my body decided that walking was just not something it was going to invest in. Most of this book shows a different side to my personality. Just remember that this part exists – and it's an important part.

My CP was diagnosed when I was 11 months old and we found out about the neuropathy when I was six years old. We've always seen these late diagnoses as a blessing in disguise because my disability wasn't the first factor influencing how my parents viewed me and what my life would or could be. Expectations existed, and when my CP was discovered, those expectations were still there – we just had to adjust the methods. Then we found out about my neuropathy, which could have been hectic. Hearing that you have something degenerative can be pretty scary, but my six-year-old self didn't understand the potential magnitude of the diagnosis. I remember going for tests a few times, but they weren't really conclusive, so from that point on we just focused on output and what I could do instead of thinking about everything that could go wrong or the function I could lose. It has been, and continues to be, a sound strategy for us.

This diagnosis didn't dictate our attitude towards my disability. What it solidified for all of us was that we have the power to focus on whatever part of my disability we want to, and we would rather focus on the ability within my disability. I believe it's important to find the positivity in situations because negativity doesn't generally lead to solutions and to reaching my goals. That's not to say that you should never be negative. I'm saying that overall positivity is helpful. I struggle with this sometimes, as let's be honest, being disabled is hard. In fact, being disabled is often really shitty.

I've realised that in order for me to find my way back to the positive, solution-oriented outlook I strive to have, sometimes you have to spend a little time just sitting in the shit. Even though there is much to be negative about, I don't want to spend all my energy in that headspace.

I can have a positive outlook while being honest about the ways my disability makes my life a mission. Choosing to be positive in the face of a lot of external negativity doesn't mean I'm naive – I fully recognise all the things that are not okay, and all the things I'm not okay with. I choose to acknowledge them and focus my energy elsewhere, on solutions. My disability has put me in some pretty ridiculous, often hilarious, situations, many of which you'll find out about later. Finding the humour in these moments is one of the strategies I use all the time to combat the negativity. Negativity isn't sustainable where there is laughter and just the right amount of sass and sarcasm.

Living with disability is such a unique experience that it can be difficult to find common ground because every disabled person is affected by their disability in different ways. This is only problematic because disabled people are placed in boxes without recognition of the massive diversity in the label "disabled". The diversity of the disabled experience leads to diversity in the challenges to be met and accommodated. There is always debate around the best approaches to solve the many challenges we each face when it comes to being a disabled person. Let's look at a "simple" example – what do you call me? There are terms that are generally accepted as not being okay to use, like handicapped. But what to say now ... disabled? Differently abled? A person with a disability? I refer to myself as all of these. (I don't feel like I have to use just one, and I don't feel like using one negates the others; I'm okay with all of these labels, so if you use these with me, you're good.) Everyone has their preferences for which labels to use and how they'd like to be referred to, so take the time to find out what people are comfortable with and go with that. I don't think it has to be so rigid as to say I have to pick one label and use it exclusively. In my opinion, the labels are not mutually exclusive and expecting me to choose one and use that forever conflicts with the diversity of disability in the first place.

Navigating disability diversity is complex; it's an ongoing journey of self-discovery and continuous learning. Balancing ideas with sensitivity is important for us to move forward to a more equal and inclusive society. As a disabled person, I also feel it's important for me to understand and interrogate, critically, why I feel the way I do about certain things. If I can understand my feelings and thoughts better, then I can be more succinct in explaining my feelings to others.

I often have to balance my feelings between gratitude and guilt. There's an idea out there that because I'm disabled, I should just be grateful. This bothers me. I am truly grateful for everything I have in my life, but there is a line. I shouldn't be expected to be grateful when I can't equitably access a building, a restaurant, transport or an education. This takes me back to a time in high school when I was at the top of a flight of stairs before the boys carried me down and I was judged as being ungrateful because I didn't appreciate a joke one of them made about pushing me down the stairs. That wasn't funny and it didn't feel like a joke to me. I was seen as being too sensitive and that I should have just been grateful that they were helping me at all. So, gratitude is complicated. I'm grateful when people help me, but I don't want to have to say thank you every time someone puts a spoonful of food in my mouth. It turns into something else then.

I think I've unintentionally internalised many of these ideas and I often worry that I am expecting too much of people and am taking up too much space, when I'm really just expecting equal treatment. I often feel guilty about asking for help all the time and expecting people around me to make a plan around my needs and to accommodate my disability in whatever activity we're doing. I do like being the centre of attention (I'm a drama queen, okay?), but sometimes I feel guilty that I *have* to be the focus when it's only because of my disability (even if it's just for a little while).

I need help with a lot of things. Most things, actually. Every morning, I wake up and I need help. I need help to change out of my pyjamas into the clothes I'll wear for that day, and to pack extra clothes into my bag in case my body rebels. Using toilets is not part of my everyday routine (I bet you're curious now!), but when I do use one, I need assistance. I can't have a shower or a bath by myself, so someone will help me with that. I can't stand or walk on my own, so I need help getting into my wheelchair. I need help putting my shoes on (when I decide I'm actually going to wear shoes), brushing my teeth, doing my hair, moisturising my face. I can't open doors or move furniture – this has to happen more often than you might think – or take things out of my bag. I need help with eating most things and I use straws for drinking.

[TANGENT]
Okay, we need to talk about straws for a minute. I'm going to try to keep this short because it has the potential of becoming a rant and it's way too early in this book for that...

All I'm going to say is: many disabled people use/need to use plastic straws because of the nature of their disability. The fact that my disability requires me to use plastic straws doesn't mean I'm against greening the planet or saving the sea turtles. I believe in these causes. I can understand the "low-hanging fruit" mentality of people stopping the use of straws, as it's the easy first step – most people don't *need* to use straws so yes, by all means refuse the plastic straw if you don't need one. The problem here is that this assumes that simply because most people don't need them, nobody needs them. It's important, though, to consider who will be affected negatively by such a movement.

We're a few years into the single-use-plastics movement and we now finally have some semi-workable alternatives to the single-use plastic straw. And even then, many disabled people can't use these alternatives because of their particular disability. Metal straws, for example, aren't great with hot drinks and if you have spasticity like I do, it's hard to close your mouth around a metal straw because it's not malleable. And silicone straws are too flexible, so they are difficult to control because of my spasticity. However, it would have been great if these solutions had been found a long time ago. For those needing to use straws this would have led to far less guilt and feeling judged for it.

We have to advocate for everything, and that can get tiring and frustrating. It means a lot when the needs of disabled people are taken into consideration when big plans to change the world are being made. Too often, disabled people have to accommodate non-disabled people's decisions or plans because there aren't enough disabled people involved or included in the discussions and decision-making processes for big movements such as the movement to eliminate single-use plastic.
[TANGENT OVER]

If you're wondering about how I would do something, I probably need some sort of assistance to get that done. I can't do a lot of things but I've learnt that doing that stuff on my own is not the most important thing in my life. There is a way to be honest about what doesn't work for me because of my disability, and still have a positive outlook on life. It's okay to have help. I can use the energy elsewhere.

I'm very much on board with doing things efficiently, even though this may seem like a contradiction when things can take decades longer than they would take a non-disabled person to do. This is where efficiency involves me having help with stuff. I can appreciate that sometimes it's good to find ways to do things for myself, and sometimes I need to delegate to save energy to do the things I've prioritised for that specific day.

My life is full (in both a scheduling sense and a feeling fulfilled sense). So no need to assume my disability has somehow left me an empty shell of a person who longs for all the things able-bodied, non-disabled living brings. We don't need that kind of energy around here. I think we still have so much work to do to combat the perceptions and stigma around disability. Too often disabled people are positioned as always needing or receiving help, resources, whatever; we need to change this narrative to look at disabled people not only as recipients but also as people capable of giving to and supporting others.

It's in the small things that my disability shows itself. I don't really think about it because it's my norm; my standard day. I live through the same number of hours as everyone else – I'm just using wheels and doing everything sitting, and I have a logistical plan for everything and three backup plans for any logistical plan.

Whenever we go anywhere, I'm always the first person to get into the car and the last to get out. Whoever is driving has to get my wheelchair into the vehicle, and if there's a group of us going, the others will be helping with that. I can tell you the boot space for most car types relative to how much of a mission it is to get a wheelchair into the boot – this is how we judge the quality of a car. Since I was about 10 years old, I've wanted to get a car that I can drive and therefore be independent. Getting a car would be incredible because it would mean that I could rely on myself to get around and I wouldn't be so dependent on other people, at least in a transport sense. It would also mean that people could rely on me for something, and that would be a great change of dynamic.

A while ago I was sitting in the car in a parking lot with my cousin Dylan, waiting for Mom to come out of a shop, and a guy parked his car in the row in front of us, got out of it and was inside the shop, all in less than 15 seconds. It was amazing to me just how easily he did all of those things; the way he probably didn't even think about the 12 things he had just done successfully to reach the shop. I didn't feel jealous. It was more a sense of awe at how quickly people can do stuff. Everything I do takes time, thought and planning.

I'm a planner, a pro-strategist, if you will. I think ahead by accident. Or maybe it's by design. Or just out of necessity. Spontaneity is hard for me, practically and emotionally. I like knowing what is happening, what's going to happen and what could happen, so that I am prepared for whatever eventuality. It can be exhausting and can make for some pretty full (and sometimes heavy) bags if you try to carry them all on your own.

I don't feel weighed down by all of these considerations and I don't want anybody to feel sorry for me because I can't do all of these things and have to have a full arsenal of backup plans. This is my reality and it has always been my reality. It's cool. I don't have a complex about my disability – I have other complexes. We'll get to those later.

My disability has definitely created challenges in my life and the lives of those around me that wouldn't exist if I were not disabled. It would be naive of me to think that it hasn't and that the world doesn't look at me differently because of my disability. And yes, sometimes it gets to me that the world can be so unaccommodating of my disability and the different ways of doing things. Even though life can be hard and overwhelming at times, I love the life I have and I'm determined to make it as profound, memorable and full as I possibly can.

I tend to talk about my disability and my body as if it were another person, not separate from myself. It's my constant partner, like a person with their own ideas, abilities, fears and perspective. Whenever I want to do something, I may want to do it in a particular way, but my disability disagrees and wants a different way or doesn't want to do it at all. Any thought I have, my disability feels the need to give its two cents' worth; whenever I need to go anywhere, my disability reminds me of the 700 things I need to remember to take with me. I'm constantly negotiating, debating or navigating situations *with* my disability. This is not a bad thing, it's just something I've realised is a reality for me. I have to decide every day whether or not I'm going to allow my disability to be the boss that day. Most days, I win the debate. It can and does get exhausting having these constant conversations with my body and sometimes I'm tired of fighting, and on those days I let my disability take a victory lap (before I gather enough energy to tell it to get back in line). I don't feel bad about this – it's all a part of being a human with a disability. This is a time where I'm embracing "people-first language", which puts a person before a diagnosis, and agree that I live with my disability and shouldn't be defined by my disability. I'm recognising my disability as an active and engaging participant in my existence, rather than something inert and disconnected that happened to me and that I now have to live with. So when I say "we" and it's not clear who I'm referring to, chances are I'm talking about myself and my disability, not myself and other people.

Stereotypes and stigma are huge barriers to proper inclusion, and one way we can combat these is to do things that counter these ideas. So, for some reason, there are those who tend to think that disabled people don't have lives like everyone else. I get looks when I'm at restaurants with friends, when I order a drink (there's more judgement when a friend orders it for me, like they're forcing me to drink), when people see I have tattoos or even when I'm just shopping.

One story that sticks with me that shocks people was when my sister, Erin, had a Sports Day at school and our family was there to support her. She was six years old or so at the time. A woman walked up to Mom, who was holding me in her arms, and said, "It's so nice that you bring her out." Why wouldn't I be there supporting my sister? Isn't that normal? This is a more common response than you might think. There are so many similar statements we encounter every day and we each have our own way of dealing with the situation.

Often people like imposing their views or their (perceived) knowledge on us. We receive a lot of unsolicited advice. When I was 12-ish I was shopping with Erin when a woman came up to us and randomly commented: "I'm an

OT, and you should tell your parents that your sister should be wearing hand splints." (Thanks for your input.)

Erin (rightly) lost her shit. I just sat back and grabbed the metaphorical popcorn because this woman was not prepared for the response she was about to receive. Erin said: "Excuse me? You don't know us. You don't know anything about our lives. My sister has been wearing all kinds of splints since she was three years old. It's the weekend; she's taking a break."

Her activism comes out in situations like this. My disability has impacted her life, but at the same time, she's not going around telling the universe that her sister has a disability – she chooses her moments. All I'm saying is, don't park in an accessible parking bay near her if you don't genuinely need it.

As I've said, I go out, I have drinks with my friends, I have multiple tattoos. It's not the biggest deal. I mean, if I were non-disabled I don't think doing these things would elicit such a response of shock and horror. I've learnt not to pay attention to this (too often) and, because it's been a feature in my life pretty much from the get-go, I don't really notice how many people are looking at me any more.

My parents are pretty cool when it comes to me living my life as I want to. As long as they know where we are and we send a location pin each time we change places, it's all good. My parents will fetch me at all hours of the night and I really appreciate this. We've always been open and able to share things with our parents, and they can't exactly say they want me to live my life and at the same time say I can't leave home after 7pm.

I have some entertaining stories that were made way more interesting by my disability. Like when a chilled birthday party turned into a night out and only when we got out of the Uber did we realise the bar we were going to was up two flights of stairs. We were less than sober at that moment. The party had started in the afternoon and it was now around 10pm. We figured out how to get upstairs and it was mostly a vibe. It wasn't the most accessible place we had chosen, but I was fine to make a plan because I didn't want to make a scene around my disability. (I choose my moments too.) So we made a plan. Leaving the bar at 1am was a bit trickier, as we were all even more inebriated than when we had arrived, so strategising took a little longer and we had more to think about. I'm still impressed that we made solid decisions that morning, considering our collective alcohol consumption. I got into an argument with a man who was trying to explain how all we needed to do was fold the chair before carrying me down the stairs. He was gesturing how to fold, as though folding up a motorised wheelchair is as simple as folding a pizza, so he annoyed me and I just told him as much. When Mom dropped me at the party, she said, "Wherever you go, the most sober person needs to carry Chaeli." We remembered this and decided that the most responsible thing to do would be to carry me separately from my chair.

Everything we were doing made complete sense, but context is important to understanding. Let me explain what people saw. I was carried down the stairs by my most sober friend, as requested by Mom, and when we got outside I was still being carried (for obvious reasons, but nobody on the pavement knew I was disabled). Mom was parked down the block in our white kombi, so we somewhat stumbled towards her, she opened the door from the inside and I was essentially tossed into the car because I was getting heavy. There was a group of women outside the entrance to the bar and when they saw us, we knew they were judging me: this girl can't hold her alcohol, can't even walk by herself… It took longer to get my wheelchair downstairs, but when it arrived on the pavement five minutes after I was shoved into a big white vehicle, the penny dropped for everyone watching. I think many lessons were learnt that evening/morning.

As for my tattoos, I started getting them when I was 16. My parents got me one for my birthday. (I told you my parents are cool.) I'd had the same idea for my first tattoo for years, and I was just waiting to be old enough to get it done. I knew I wanted to have it between my shoulder blades and I wanted to get the Chinese symbol for resilience. At the time of getting that tattoo I was having a tough time at school, so it made sense to me in the moment but would also be relevant for me going forward. I now have a number of tattoos and each one is important to me. They aren't on my body to make a point to anyone else. Each one has a special meaning and reminds me of a specific time in my life when I learnt some hard lessons, and when I see them I can go back to those moments and find strength. I look at them and am proud that those experiences have made me who I am today. In my view, my tattoos are a part of my story and having the ability to express myself through my body is not always possible because of my disability. So, I'm claiming power and agency over my body through these pieces of art and storytelling.

I'm open about my disability and its effect on my life. It can be complicated but it can also be simple. It has always been a priority for me to have good communication around my disability, and with others. Eye contact has always been a crucial part of how I engage with people around me. This can also be complicated because, being in a wheelchair, I am practically shorter than others and this leads to some negotiating on my part, to make sure that I'm able to engage meaningfully with whoever I'm talking to... I'm very happy for you to pull up a chair to have a chat. I love engaging with people – I believe that by talking to one another we can get closer to a deeper understanding of each of our perspectives. When I was little, I would sit on the counter in our kitchen so that I could be a part of the conversation instead of being on the floor looking at people's knees or in my wheelchair looking at people's belly buttons. This helped me establish where I should place myself and how I should expect to be seen and treated in my everyday life.

RELATIONSHIPS CHANGE EVERYTHING

I feel lucky to have been born into the family I have. I have incredible parents who have always expected things of me. This is big. I was never allowed to use my disability as an excuse not to get involved and live my life. While being disabled has clearly impacted my life in hugely significant ways, I don't see it as the core defining feature of my existence. I was always encouraged to try new things and have experiences just as anybody else would or should.

My dad, Russell, is an only child and has lived in Cape Town his whole life, while my mom, Zelda, is one of six children and grew up in Welkom in the Free State. She's convinced that wherever we go, whoever we meet, she can find a Welkom connection. It's ridiculous how accurate this is. She says that the only thing that changes is the amount of time it takes to find that connection.

My mom is probably the most epic human I know. She is a force to be reckoned with, and when she walks into a room, her presence is known. She has always been determined to help me live a life of meaning and she will often say to me, "Chaeli, my role is to challenge you." My mom is passionate about changing the world and is a total optimist. We spend most of our time together. Our relationship is special and we're lucky to have the opportunity to have such a close bond. We don't really have to say anything out loud because we know what the other is thinking. I know that my activist streak has come from her and we spend long road trips strategising how we can make the world more inclusive and ranting that "Surely it isn't that hard?" but in the same breath saying how complicated it is to live in this world and solve these problems.

My dad has a quiet power, which is cool. He just prefers to be behind the scenes. Dad's got some interesting hobbies and when he discovers something interesting, he will find out everything about it and that knowledge gets passed on to us. So if I have ever come out with a random piece of information (like what a particular word is in Morse code or how to communicate through radio in a crisis), now you know, it came from my popsicle. He loves his family fiercely and is ready to take people on if they've treated any of us unfairly. Every so often my dad's activist side comes out – he's sort of an undercover activist. His activist side is powerful because it's unexpected and he often sees things differently, so it makes you think about the issue from a different perspective.

I have one sibling, an older sister, Erin, who always keeps me grounded and holds me accountable for using my ability as much as I can. This often annoys me because sometimes I'm just tired and sometimes it's nice to be helped, but I also appreciate the reminder. Sometimes. Older sisters are great advice-givers and sounding boards. Erin is 15 months older than me and she owns this fact, just as many older siblings do. She can be overprotective and totally frustrates me when she wants to be the boss, but I value her input and I don't know what I would do without her in my life. We shared a room until I was 13 years old, and then we needed our own space. We made some awesome memories through sharing a bedroom – all the late-night conversations, laughs and being yelled at to go to sleep because we were being too loud. One slightly problematic outcome of sharing a room is that my sister became "immune" to my calls at night (when I need to turn over, or I'm getting hot, or a mosquito bites me and I'm itchy), so when the two of us are travelling together and sharing a room, I need to be loud or nudge her awake. We've totally worked it out, though. I think it may be better now that she has children; she's tuned in differently now that she's a mom.

I'm obsessed with my nephews – they are the most gorgeous humans. I know I have aunt bias, but I truly believe they are gorgeous from an objective point of view. It's amazing to see them grow and learn about disability as they grow. They make me believe that inclusion is definitely possible: they've been embracing it their entire lives. Since birth they have just absorbed the fact that I do things differently, so they work differently with me than with their parents. When Erin once asked her first-born (Mom calls Erin this all the time too) "Can Aunty Chaeli walk?" he looked at her as if she made no sense, matter-of-factly responded "No" and swiftly moved on to playing a different game, completely unfazed. He has never seen me walk and he knows my wheelchair is my means of getting around. The boys know that they have to ask if they want to ride on my chair, and they know that if they want to play with me, they need to find a way to reach me. And they always make a plan to do just that.

When Erin's husband, Warren, came into our lives I was excited to have a brother. I like having an older brother and it feels as though he's always been part of our family. Warren is one of the most supportive people I've ever known. He is always ready to take on new challenges and often says, "There are no problems, only solutions." When I met him for the first time I was taken aback because he understood what I was saying right from the start, whereas many people struggle with this because of my speech impediment and I often need to repeat myself. When I asked him why it was so easy for him to understand me (insert internalised ableism here), he said, "You just have a different accent. And I listen." Ha. So simple. In some ways, introducing people to me and seeing how they engage with me has been a sort of litmus test for my sister, and Warren passed that one with flying colours. He's also great at making tea, and that's always a bonus.

I wasn't surrounded by disability from the moment I arrived on this Earth. Most of the time I wasn't, and this is still the case today. We weren't even exposed to my own disability until I was almost a year old. In my everyday life, my initial friend circle was non-disabled, and I think that's a good indication of what life is like when you have a disability, whatever that disability may be. It can be hard to find other disabled people to associate with and be friends with. I think disability can be very isolating a lot of the time. Being disabled is not a recognised standard in society, even though there are a lot of disabled people in the world – if you have a disability you're not seen as "normal" and often society expects less of you because of it. I choose to hold myself to a higher standard than society's expectations of me, and it is not by chance that I have this attitude. I have family and friends (who are also basically family) who have never treated me as being "less than" because I'm disabled. My family have encouraged and taught those around us to see me as capable and for me that is an unbelievable gift that I am constantly reminded of – every time someone tells me I can't do something because I'm disabled; every time someone leans in uncomfortably close and changes their pitch or volume when they speak to me; every time I receive gazes with furrowed brows and pitying eyes; every time I get to a set of stairs without an accessible alternative – because my understanding of myself or self-worth is not created or dictated by these moments and perceptions. Instead it is built on a sense of optimism and self-worth that acts as my armour against the negative ideas.

Family and friends have played a huge part in how I've defined myself and my disability. I'm grateful that the people around me have always made plans around my disability and don't make it a huge deal. Our family are lucky to have lifelong friends in the Terry sisters – Tarryn, Justine and Chelsea. To be honest, we didn't have much of a choice in building our friendship. Our parents became friends at the Bergvliet Sports Association, or the sports club, as we call it, before we all existed and when we arrived they basically told us to play nicely together. I'm glad it worked out and we ended up liking one another. We're such a ridiculous crew and obviously we have our days when we irritate one another and fight about stupid things, but it's great to have friends who have been around forever and you know they're going to be around when life gets a little too real to handle alone. We are more like family than friends; we still spend every Christmas together and it's just the best day ever.

When we were little, Tarryn, Justine, Chelsea, Erin and I would spend hours dismantling my wheelchair into its smallest possible pieces. We always felt that we needed to be completely ready to be self-sufficient with wheelchair mechanics should the day ever come when we might need these skills and nobody else was around to help us out.

When other kids wanted to play with me they would often ask Mom if they could. And even now people still ask her (or anyone else who is with me) questions rather than me – in restaurants when we are ordering food, or when people are just curious about my life and they have questions. My mom always used to say, "Well, ask Chaeli" because maybe I didn't want to play with them; maybe they weren't cool people – and by that I mean "nice", not "cool" as in having social status – and I didn't want to be around them. Autonomy and making decisions for myself have clearly been important since the beginning. There were also always expectations, of me and those around me... "If you want to play with Chaeli then you need to do a few things." First, we needed to make sure it was a game that I could play, and if it wasn't we had to change the rules of the game or find a new way to include me in the game. For example, when we were playing cricket I would be the umpire, and when I played soccer with my cousins when we were on holiday I would be the goalkeeper.

[TANGENT]
There was much more strategy to this than we were given credit for as 10-year-olds. The plan was twofold. We figured that because I was in a wheelchair, on a practical level I would take up the most space in the goal. And then on a more psychological level, we embraced the prejudice of other people thinking that I was a fragile porcelain doll, and they wouldn't want to kick a soccer ball at full speed into the face of a kid in a wheelchair. Both parts of this strategy were effective, until the other kids worked out that we were playing them. It worked for one holiday trip, and then we had to find new winning strategies after that.
[TANGENT OVER]

We would also simply create new games. One of these was a game called *Boo Ya!* (I've clarified with the co-creators that this was in fact the name.) I guess it was an adapted form of football or goalball, where we used a long neck pillow instead of a ball. (If you get hit in the face with a neck pillow it's a lot less dangerous and there's lower risk of someone calling the parents.) The game was played on mattresses in our lounge and the try zone was on either side of the edge of the mattresses. I think we were only allowed to move if someone else helped you move. This is not necessarily a team game. It was always difficult to play games that required teams because we were five people, but in *Boo Ya!* (patent pending) the rule was that we had teams of two and then the leftover person could decide whichever team they felt like supporting in that moment.

So, we had the first rule sorted, the "be creative with your games". The second rule was that everyone had to remember not to leave me on my own when the game location moved. If people forgot about rule two, then rule three would come into effect: "If you forget Chaeli somewhere, you're going to get moaned at and you'll be sufficiently reminded of the importance of rule two." I was only forgotten or left somewhere a few times, but it never took them long to remember they had forgotten about me. I learnt forgiveness early in life. This rule was only applicable until I got my motorised wheelchair (when I was nine). There were a few times that we deliberately didn't listen to this rule, like when we were playing hide-and-seek.

On one occasion we were playing hide-and-seek at the sports club and we found a really good hiding place for me and Chelsea, I think it was. We thought it would be funny to hide in a different spot from where my wheelchair was to confuse the opposition (come to think of it, this could also be a sound strategy in a zombie apocalypse), so we left my wheelchair inside and we hid in the hedge next to the tennis courts. We felt successful because we were there for quite a while, so we thought we were winning. We won that round but quickly realised that it was probably not such a great hiding place when we couldn't figure out how to get me out of the hedge. We were stuck. The rest of the group went to find a rescue team, namely David, another family friend who is also the general manager of the Bergvliet Sports Association. He was also the least likely to yell at us for putting ourselves in such a situation. When he arrived he asked us how we got in there in the first place. Our response was something like, "We just did it!" Anything is possible when someone's counting to 30. I'm pretty sure this story ended with David cutting us out of the hedge like a firefighter. It was then agreed that I should probably stay in my wheelchair for the duration of this game. Probably a smart move.

We have so many stories just like this. Many people have similar stories and that's awesome; that's what life's about. Keep living your life and share those stories in whatever way you want. I've learnt that my disability has definitely added a special layer of storytelling to my life.

I'm grateful that I have been allowed to try things, to make mistakes and to get hurt. This may sound hectic, but it happens. Children fall regularly and they learn from each of these experiences. I don't see why I should be denied this learning experience because I'm disabled and in a wheelchair.

Many people may think it's reckless or somewhat irresponsible of my parents to leave me, an objectively severely disabled and vulnerable child, in the hands of a group of relatively responsible children. However, you need to realise that we always knew when things were getting to be too much for us and would then call an adult to help us. I truly appreciate that I don't have helicopter parents who stick so close to me that I don't have a life outside of them. I've been allowed to be my own person, make decisions and have experiences where I've learnt valuable life lessons, and the people I've shared these experiences with have learnt these too, alongside a few extra ones. Is this a "riskier" life? Definitely. I wouldn't trade it, though, because in all of the madness, creative game changes, bad decisions, injuries and shedding of tears (happy and sad ones) are shared life experiences and stories that we can tell our children and anybody else who'll listen. They're proof that I've lived, and am still living, a life that is good and *full*!

That is what we all hope for, isn't it?

We joke a lot about how inconvenient my disability can be, and there is a lot of honesty behind these jokes, but it doesn't mean that acknowledging how admin-heavy my life is, is necessarily being negative about being disabled. We have to acknowledge it so that we can tackle it in a meaningful way, while still remaining sane and positive about how we can contribute to society and leave a legacy, and live a life that makes a difference to other people. We cannot just live and exist for ourselves, we have to share ourselves with the world because our stories are worth sharing. I think I have a good one so far, and I'm working on adding to the craziness. I'll continue to share it with those around me and we'll learn together.

When I began my investigations into getting a service dog, I wasn't old enough to get one, but the desire stayed with me. I researched it from the time I was about 10 years old. In South Africa there are only a few organisations training them, and each has a specific niche market it caters for. I found the South African Guide-Dogs Association for the Blind, which provides working dogs for people with mobility impairments, so I kept track. I was in high school when I eventually applied for a service dog and I knew they had quite a long waiting list to receive one of these stellar creatures. I applied and obsessed over it, coming up with strategies for integrating my yet-to-be-given service dog into my life, but after a few months it slipped off my radar.

While I was on the waiting list the trainers did various interviews to see whether I was suitable to be a service-dog owner and to clarify which skills my dog would need so that they wouldn't do any training for unnecessary skills.

It's a lengthy process. To have a working dog you need puppies, and they have to grow and develop and learn proper skills, so it takes some time. Many of the puppies are not suited to a life of service and that can only be determined later, so there's a fair amount of wait and see. The skills a service dog needs to master depend on their person's disability, as well as the lifestyle they lead. Dogs have personalities just as people do, and this is taken into consideration too. The South African Guide-Dogs Association for the Blind takes the matching process extremely seriously, as it should. It's probably one of the most important aspects to having a successful working-dog team. I have learnt that there is so much happening behind the scenes when you're thinking there is nothing going on. It's hard to be on the receiving end of this process because you don't hear anything until a dog is ready for you. My friends say that my pup is the canine version of me, so I reckon they did a great job with the matching process.

I don't believe in coincidence and I know everything happens when it needs to. My parents were speaking, just hypothetically, about whether we should get more animals. But service dogs are not pets, so that solved that dilemma. (That's what I call a loophole.) Two weeks after this hypothetical conversation I was notified that there was a dog for me, and she would be ready for me in a month or so. Her name was Eden, a yellow Labrador retriever.

I was *so* excited! I immediately started looking for her on all of the South African Guide-Dogs Association for the Blind's social media accounts, but they don't post names on the dogs' pictures (probably for this exact reason). It's important that people don't get attached to any of the dogs prematurely. I justified my obsession, saying that they had told me that Eden was mine, so I was just searching for evidence of her existence. I was only given one photograph of her sitting inside an office, so it wasn't a lot to go on. Eventually I stopped looking and just waited for the day that I'd get to meet her. Together with all of the excitement was the realisation of the responsibility involved in getting a service dog. I was about to become a mom to this pup – her forever person – and I was going to be her go-to person, her safe place. Little did I know she would become mine too.

She arrived on a Saturday – 18 October 2014. I was so nervous and excited and all kinds of other emotions. I knew it was a life-changing day. Eden arrived at our front gate and as we opened it there were so many expectations from all sides. She was at the house for about two minutes when her trainer, Leon, undid her leash to allow her to explore her new home. Not even 30 seconds later, Eden spotted our swimming pool and decided it required investigating. She did a less than graceful but enthusiastic swan dive into the water! Leon said they didn't know she would react that way to swimming pools and apologised profusely. When they asked her puppy raiser, Bonnie (the person she stayed with for the first year or so of her life before she started her official, specific-skills training), about it, she explained it down to the smallest detail. I think maybe Eden knew that it was a tense situation, and someone had to break the tension, so she decided it should be her. Everyone was a lot more chilled after that, so I guess it worked.

While Eden went exploring, Leon explained some things about her personality and what the training process entailed. He passed me a present and a letter. They were from Bonnie. I read the letter and it was beautiful. She explained that Eden is a feisty one and has been from the start. (Eden is the baby of a litter of nine, so she's clearly a fighter.) Bonnie shared the story of how, when Eden was a puppy, she found her sitting in the footwell of her new car (this is her place), very quietly and determinedly chewing her way through the airbag mechanism. She could have killed herself. It's just like little kids – if they're unusually quiet, it's time to worry because they're probably getting up to no good! Erin helped me to unwrap the present, and it was a collage of photos of baby Eden. This was a really thoughtful gift and it means a lot to me – service-dog owners don't experience that part of their pup's life. When we get them, they arrive with skills, ready to work. It was special that Bonnie had given us a small part of that journey. Sometimes I get a little bit of FOMO, because we don't get to see or love them from when they're babies, but then I remember the airbag story, and all the work and stress that goes into raising puppies, and then I'm okay with it.

Puppy raisers are a special breed of humans. They open their homes and hearts to these cute little puppies with purpose, love them and work with them for a year, and when the pups are ready they let them go to live out their life of service. It's just incredible.

I eased into the role of service-dog owner. Eden came down from Johannesburg and stayed at the Cape Town offices for the weekend; she would come home for good on the Monday. Leon contacted us on Monday morning and asked us to meet with him that afternoon because he needed to share something with us. I was instantly stressed, thinking that something terrible had happened. Always one to think of the worst circumstance first, I thought she had contracted some crazy Cape Town-based disease and was dying. Cue the overly dramatic, protective new dog mom. When we met up with Leon, Eden wasn't with him. So naturally, I thought, "I was right." Turns out, on Saturday after our meeting, Eden had had an encounter with a cat. (She didn't attack it or anything, she just got too excited and wanted to play with it – the cat wasn't on board and ran away.) This encounter had triggered a seizure. Leon told us that she was fine, and the vet determined that Eden has epilepsy. Exhale, everybody.

Leon offered us a choice. We could keep Eden or we could give her back and wait for another dog without any issues. If we chose the latter, there would be no judgement. He told us that her epilepsy was totally manageable and, when managed, it wouldn't affect her ability to perform her tasks as a service dog. Clearly I decided to keep her. Even though I had only known her for a number of hours, she was mine. I knew in my heart that she was mine, regardless of any challenges she would face. Also, what message would that be sending about my activism, if we found out Eden had a disability and sent her back? I had waited four years for her, and they had determined we were a perfect match. It was a no-brainer – we were used to baggage, so we would just get some more suitcases to carry Eden's too. Decision made.

I went on a research mission to find out as much as I could about epilepsy in dogs, and training commenced. In case you're wondering, epilepsy is pretty much the same for all species. We manage Eden's with medication and she's 100%. Every so often her medication needs adjusting because her body gets used to it. I've learnt the triggers and we try to avoid those.

We did Eden's training in my real-life schedule. People usually go to the training centre for a few weeks for focused training, but I was in the middle of exam prep and couldn't do that, so we adjusted the plan.

Eden is a pup of many talents, but there are definitely limits. She is still a dog. Someone asked me whether I would still need my personal-care assistant when I got Eden. Well, how do you think Eden is going to put my jeans on me? (I'm sure you can picture my face when this happened.) In these moments I generally stay quiet and wait for people to realise the error of their ways...

To clarify, Eden helps me with tasks that are often taken for granted – picking up things I drop; opening and closing doors; pressing lift buttons (and light switches when they're low enough); making a scene (by barking when I say "speak") to alert people to the fact that I need help or I'm stuck somewhere. And no, she doesn't press individual lift buttons, she presses all of them! So you just make sure you've allotted enough time to stop on every level. If there are people around or with me, it's totally okay for them to assist me. It doesn't negate Eden's purpose. She's not sensitive about it.

Many people don't realise Eden is a service dog with very specific skills because she doesn't actively practise them every moment of the day. She does get vocal sometimes, but that's just her inner activist. She spends a lot of her time sleeping next to me, snoring. I'm used to her snoring like a 90-year-old with sleep apnoea, so I don't really hear it any more. I only notice it when other people react to it, for instance when our politics lecturer would make a comment like, "Well, I guess I need to make my lectures more interesting." (We tended to agree. We appreciated Eden communicating how we were feeling, and nobody could get upset because she was just sleeping.) When people start looking around in the library to see who is passed out on a desk but see no-one, it's Eden – discreetly positioned under my desk – getting her beauty sleep. I guess it's not as discreet as I thought.

Eden has done and still does so much more than this for me. Much of what she does for me is not in the tasks she's trained to do, it's in everything else.

She is endlessly committed and loyal. As I'm writing, she's sitting at my feet, with her face touching my front wheel. It's where she belongs; wherever we are, whether she's attached to me or not, whether she's in work mode or not, she is right there with some part of her body connected to me. The cutest is when she puts her face on my feet, staring up at me with her very convincing puppy-dog eyes. People can't handle it. I embrace this sometimes, but I can totally resist it when she's trying to be manipulative. Although she tries to push the boundaries regularly, which is understandable, she definitely knows when she needs to be on her best behaviour, representing the entire canine workforce. She is impeccable in any sort of official place – in a bank, in a hospital, at the airport. So good. It just proves that she does understand expectations and boundaries. I rest my case.

You may have some burning questions about service-dog travel logistics... When we're in a car, she sits in the footwell at my feet. If I'm on a bus or something, she'll be next to me just like when I'm sitting at a desk. Yes, you can travel on planes with working dogs, as long as you have all of the required and up-to-date documents for them. No, they don't go in a crate into the hold – they sit at your feet so they can be helpful. Whenever I have flown with Eden, the pilots have been in awe of her – as they should be – and most of the time, Eden has been the flight crew's first working dog on board. She just sleeps and occasionally digs her nails into the floor if there's turbulence and for take-off and landing.

Now, my Eden is very intuitive and it's unbelievable the way she can sniff out someone who needs a little bit of love or just some recognition. I think this is partly why many people mistake her for an emotional-support dog. She was not officially trained with any skills to be an emotional-support dog, but she's gained on-the-job training. I struggle with anxiety, which has become more of a thing in my life in the past few years (and especially now, as we wade our way through a global pandemic). I realised my pup has some hidden talents when I had an intense panic attack in a stairwell on campus during my honours year. In a nutshell, we weren't able to reach my seminar venue because none of the lifts was working. I had so many thoughts running through my mind and I didn't know what to do. I was crying and hyperventilating, and Eden sprang into action. Her response to any kind of negative stress from humans is excessive happiness. She sees that I'm struggling and moves into position (on my left side). She starts wagging her tail like crazy, jumps up, puts her front paws on the table of my chair and licks my face so much that I get distracted from my panic. She's done this for a few of my friends too.

I've heard a lot of working-dog owners say that you get the dog you need. I didn't really understand what this meant, but I'm starting to. Having Eden in my life has led to so many moments of joy, empowerment and self-discovery.

I have always believed in my ability to be independent and seen myself as a confident, competent person. I didn't realise how much of the world's external pressure of being a self-sufficient person weighs on me and how I do things. It took me a while to be okay with asking Eden to do things for me because I had always found strategies to do them on my own. I had to trust and accept that she is also an acceptable strategy partner in navigating the world. With her around, I don't have to reserve so much brain space for planning for "What if I drop something?" or "How am I going to get into that room if the door is closed?" These may seem like small things, but these thoughts or questions have kept me from being present in a space or experience on many occasions. Yes, I now have to remember to take her outside regularly to go "busy-busy" and make sure she has water and is happy, but that is much simpler to deal with than the constant stress and panic about tiny things most people don't even notice. Eden brings a sense of peace in those moments. She has enabled me to accept people's eyes more willingly. I mean, I've always embraced people's eyes because they've always been a presence in my life, but now, with Eden at my side, I can sometimes assume they're directed in her direction. People have a more positive look on their faces when they watch us and it's not just, "Oh shame, she's disabled. Her life must be so tough." Now it's more, "Oh look, she has a dog." She makes me feel less disabled, less judged. I feel more empowered when she's around.

Eden has definitely given me more confidence to speak up. I'm not sure if it's just because she projects a level of sass and attitude that's rubbing off on me. Maybe it's that I have to use my voice with conviction when I work with her, so I take myself more seriously because she does; maybe it's that I have to speak up for her when people are being idiots around her. I know her best and I'm her protector. That's not a role I'm used to, having a disability (I'm generally seen more on the vulnerable group side of society), so it's been a journey to discover that side of myself. My mama bear instincts can kick in pretty strongly if you're being an asshole to my bub.

Eden has so many sides to her personality and it's been amazing to uncover them. When she is dressed in her work jacket she is a professional. She loves working. She is also super playful when "off-duty" and runs around like a mad thing, but is also totally happy to do nothing and just take a five-hour nap. She fits so well with me. She's complex and I love it.

I know she will retire at some point, and I'll get another pup. She can teach the newbie the ropes and how I work. That pup will bring their own unique gifts and lessons to my life, and that will be a whole experience, but it's one of the inevitable things in the life of a service-dog owner. I know that someday she won't be here and that's hard to think about. I hope that when it happens, she's happy and feels fulfilled with her life and career. For now, though, I'm embracing everything she is and the light she is in our lives. On Eden's first birthday with me, I posted a birthday celebration photo and Bonnie wrote a comment that hit my heart, hard. It said, "Eden was born to be with you." I ugly-cried for 10 minutes after I read that because I truly believe this. She's been my first soulmate and she's a part of me now. I'm so grateful for every part of her journey that led to her being mine.

My life lens is one with disability – there's no getting around this. It's a fact of my life.

I have always been encouraged to engage with people when they looked curious or asked questions about my disability, especially when it was kids my own age. A lot of the time people don't know what to do or say around me. They're uncomfortable. I love it when kids come up to me with questions because there's no malice in their curiosity, no judgement; they just need to know, and once they've received the information they move on. Adults complicate these interactions because they tend to overthink things and feel self-conscious and embarrassed that they don't know things, and try to make as though they haven't noticed that I'm disabled, even more so when their children disregard expected social norms and ask disabled strangers personal questions. I love that. It's pure, honest curiosity.

"What's wrong with your legs?"

"Why do your hands look like that?"

Since I was able to talk, I was taught to respond and answer questions like this:

"There's nothing wrong with me; I was made this way. I just use my body differently."

These could have been negative moments for me, where I felt made fun of, but questions were framed positively as an opportunity to educate someone with information and knowledge based on my lived experience. Having a script of sorts on hand was a helpful and simple way that I was empowered to own my disability, and the pre-planned response ensured it wasn't a stressful situation, as I knew what to say. It's okay to talk about disability without it being confrontational. Even though it was framed positively in my life, we should acknowledge that from the beginning I had to be armed with strategies to prove my worth to others and to find words to validate my existence in the world, just because I navigate the world differently.
[TANGENT]

Here's the first taste of the complicated spectrum of feelings about being disabled. My path has been one of embracing the activist side to disability, but that's not everybody's path and that's valid. It isn't my job, every waking moment, to make sure non-disabled people have an understanding of what disabled life is. If I choose to share, that's cool, and if I choose not to share my experiences, that's cool too. It becomes an issue when non-disabled people expect us to share without considering our perspective and/or how sharing may impact the disabled person.

So for me, being an activist is a part of my makeup as a person. If I weren't disabled, I fully believe I'd still be an activist. It's in my soul. I think my disability has given me a unique position and experience to be "activisty" about.
[TANGENT OVER]

In this way, I believe I have always been an activist. Activism is often rooted in personal experience and personal struggles, and my story is no different. Activism came into my life out of necessity. There was no "aha" moment when I decided I was going to be an activist. I saw how the people around me, my family and friends, would advocate for me, and I learnt early on that if I wanted to access all of my rights and do the things my friends were doing, I had to find and use my voice to make it happen.

The first big lesson in this came when I was two years old. I didn't have any balance, and if I was sitting on the floor and someone came too close to me, I'd panic, fall over and cry, feeling very sorry for my tiny, helpless self. I have a vague recollection of this happening. Mom tells me that on one occasion she sat my self-pitying self up, had a serious conversation with me about the things I had going for me, and said it was time to use them.

"You have a voice. You know when someone is making you uncomfortable or unsafe, like you're going to fall. When that happens, use your voice, make it loud and say, 'No!'"

It was not okay for me to just lie down and view myself as a victim who couldn't do anything about my situation. I had power and I had to claim it. This is how we have always approached my disability and I've taken lessons like this into my adult life, advocating for inclusion and access for myself and other disabled people.

The world could definitely be more accessible than it is – buildings, transport, experiences, everything. While there should be accessibility in all spaces, many times we're told that it's not possible or viable (economically) to make it accessible because there aren't enough disabled people who make use of inaccessible places. It's a self-fulfilling cycle of inaccessibility: no access means no disabled people, and no disabled people means no reason to create access. I think this is one instance where "build it (and make it accessible) and they will come" applies.

Inaccessibility is a surmountable barrier. I'm not saying it's okay that places are not accessible to disabled people – they should be. But I don't take a hard line of not going into a building unless I can access it completely independently. I don't believe this to be an effective method of raising awareness. I don't want to exclude myself. I don't really check whether places we're going to are accessible before we go there. (I probably should, just to be prepared for a fight, if necessary.) If a place is not accessible, we make a plan and, occasionally, we make a scene. If I have to be assisted to get in somewhere – carried up some stairs, for example – that's a memorable experience for the people who help me, and next time they walk up those stairs without a 60kg wheelchair, they are hopefully more aware.

My activism strategies are experiential; sharing stories and taking time to speak through challenges and misunderstandings to find common ground. Connecting as individuals, disabled or otherwise, has powerful implications for how it is possible to live inclusively.

I live my activism every day because I do what I want. I know that saying it in this way seems to oversimplify the issues I face as a disabled person, but sometimes it *is* this simple. I occupy unexpected spaces and I do unexpected things, like doing ultramarathons and climbing mountains, and getting multiple degrees. Every time I do something like this I'm challenging the perceptions and preconceived ideas of what disabled people "should" be doing.

I'm 100% fine with confusing people into a state of awareness.

THE CHAELI CAMPAIGN

Keeping everything you've read up until now in mind, let's look at the origin story, work and ethos behind our non-profit organisation, The Chaeli Campaign, and how it has changed our lives and the lives of the people it supports.

Remember, I got my first wheelchair when I was three years old. Before then I was carried everywhere.

[TANGENT]
You know what annoys me a lot? When people say I'm wheelchair-bound. There are a lot of ways people label me with my disability, but this one gets to me. Wheelchairs are not negative things. They are a tool of empowerment because without a wheelchair, my life would be a thousand times more difficult and less interesting. If I don't have a wheelchair, I'm far less able to do stuff, so calling me wheelchair-bound makes it sound like a wheelchair is the worst thing to be attached to. Wheelchairs are wonderful, life-changing devices.

Stop saying these things. Please?!
[TANGENT OVER]

When I was nine years old, we went to CE Mobility in Maitland in Cape Town to get my wheelchair fixed because one of the wheels had fallen off. While I was there I noticed a "Chaeli-sized" motorised wheelchair. I had a quick ride around the showroom – and I was in love. Being able to decide for myself where I wanted to go or be was a huge deal. I didn't want to get out of the wheelchair. The chair was expensive and we couldn't afford it. Seeing my enthusiasm, Martha, the manager, suggested that we sell cookies or something to raise the funds. I don't think any of us realised the seed that was planted that day, and what it would grow into.

After a few hours of thinking and discussing ideas with Erin, Tarryn, Justine and Chelsea, we came up with a plan. We were going to raise enough money to buy a motorised wheelchair, so that I could have more independence. We decided that we would sell cards and DIY plant-your-own-sunflower kits (we called them Sunshine Pots), and take orders for Saturday morning muffins, because who can say no to Saturday morning muffins? We only made the muffins for one weekend because it was a lot of effort and we enjoyed sleeping too much, so the plan was adapted slightly. In our brainstorming we had consulted just a little with our grown-ups, who didn't think we were as serious as we were about the project, but we weren't deterred. We were excited about our new mission. We had done random stuff before in school holidays, but we hadn't involved outside people. We had a clear goal (R20 000 for a motorised wheelchair) and we were determined to reach it, however long it took.

On our first day of sales we walked around our neighbourhood. The only negative encounter we had (which ended up being a positive one for us) was when we rang the doorbell of an old man who wasn't interested in supporting us in any way. He saw us as pesky kids and grumpily asked, "If I give you R5, will you go away?" We weren't disheartened. It was still early in the day and there were plenty more houses to visit. We negotiated him up to R10 and wished him a great day. We had just made money with basically no effort and we hadn't had to give him any products. We viewed that as a win.

The response from the community was unbelievable and we made R280 that day. We were thrilled. We were on our way to meeting our target!

Our original plan was to sell our products at our school's Market Day, which was happening in a couple of months' time. We didn't want to lose momentum or the excitement we had, and Mom suggested that we speak to our principal to see if we could involve our school in a more meaningful way and to ask if we could share our mission with all the pupils, take orders and have people collect their orders on Market Day. He said yes and organised a box in the foyer in which people could place their order forms. We sent order forms to everyone and waited to see what would happen.

We were blown away when we went to collect them the following day. As we opened the box, order forms spilled out all over the floor. There were hundreds of orders – far more than we had expected. We took them home to tally how many cards and Sunshine Pots we needed to make and deliver. We had to make *thousands*! Sunshine Pots and cards, we discovered, are admin-intensive items to make and it became clear that it was too much for us to do on our own, so we called in reinforcements. My Grade 4 class and our teacher (who now works with us at The Chaeli Campaign as principal of our Pre-School and Enrichment Centre – see, once you're in the family it's hard to leave) came to my house over the weekend and we had a "work party".

There were too many Sunshine Pots to deliver them all on one day, so we organised to deliver them to our school in the weeks leading up to Market Day. This turned out to be a good move, as a number of people who saw the pots at school before Market Day bought them. We never expected that we would reach our R20 000 target so quickly. We had raised the funds in seven weeks! It was such an incredible feeling to have so much support and to see everyone come together to make our goal a reality. It was the most epic crowdfunding I've ever personally experienced and been a part of.

The experience taught all of us what can happen when communities come together to help one another. It taught us the importance of being there for your friends. It taught us that you can start small and simple, with clarity and conviction, and if you have these things, goals become so much easier to achieve. And it taught us, a group of girls between the ages of six and 12, that we shouldn't listen to people who tell us we can't do things, or that our dreams are too big or too unrealistic. We proved them wrong.

I got my wheelchair and it was one of the most exciting days of my life. For the first time I was in complete control of my movement. We were still on a buzz and in a state of disbelief, but also contented because we had achieved what we had set out to do, and much faster than we'd anticipated. We had expected it to take years, but I'm so happy it didn't take that long. A while after we thought we'd wrapped up the whole Chaeli Campaign idea as a successful project, people who had bought from us came back wanting more cards or Sunshine Pots, and someone donated a second-hand adult motorised wheelchair.

We weren't sure what to do. We had reached our goal; what were we meant to do with this money and the wheelchair? The answer was simple. We needed to find other people to support. We needed to channel the goodwill and community *gees* (meaning "spirit" in Afrikaans) we had inspired and pay it forward. People connected with the simplicity of what we were doing, and I think with the fact that our work was rooted in friendship and love.

So, our first beneficiary (apart from me) was Vanessa, who has spina bifida. We raised funds for a wheelchair for her so that she could also have more independence. This was the beginning of a journey that has introduced us to some rad humans and taken us to some epic places. The wheelchair that was donated found its home with a young man, Gareth, who stayed at Woodside Special Care Centre in Rondebosch.

We formalised our work into a non-profit organisation to enable us to support so many more disabled people. Mom became CEO and Di (Mom to Tarryn, Justine and Chelsea, and "Aunty Mom" to Erin and me) became the financial manager. Together our moms make a phenomenal team and have done an incredible job of guiding our organisation over the past 17 years. We agreed that the five of us who started The Chaeli Campaign would remain involved in whatever way possible. Our main job at that time was school (we weren't even teens at that stage...). By the time we officially launched, we had already supported six disabled children to get wheelchairs specially fitted for them. We had a big celebration at Kelvin Grove Club in Newlands and it was special because our first six beneficiaries celebrated with us at the event. It was a big deal for us that they were included in that moment.

Fast-forward 17 years and we're still here. I'm super happy about that! We now have the opportunity to support between 7 000 and 9 000 people annually through our various programmes. I've been able to travel all over the world advocating for disability rights, which is amazing. Our work has grown and evolved in interesting and organic ways. The organisation has essentially grown up with us.

Our programmes started simple, focusing on providing disabled children with specialised assistive devices. It has always been crucial for us to know the people we help, as we want to know their stories and connect meaningfully. Then, as we grew, we developed more programmes like Therapies and Inclusive Education, guided by our experiences of my disability, the needs I've had and what has been important for me to access a full life. Now, we focus more on advocacy and awareness-raising because we believe that to empower disabled people, we also need to empower the people and communities around them. Ultimately, we believe that this will have a stronger impact and lead to more inclusive communities.

We've learnt some big lessons as we've grown and we have used these in our work going forward. As I mentioned earlier, we love getting to know people and supporting them at different levels (people tend to have more than a single need in their lives) and we invest in them. It's important to us to build strong relationships and recognise the humanity of each person we work with. We don't want to dictate how people should live their lives, so we tell them about the different ways we can support them. It's then up to them to let us know what they need from us, and we go from there. Meeting people in their time of need is a big deal, especially when you have a disability. So often choices are taken away from us, or decisions are made for us by other people. It's empowering when our right to choose and our right to self-determination are recognised and respected.

Advocacy and being an activist is definitely not an easy road. It's emotional; it's exhausting. I highly recommend it, though. It's totally worth it. Every person deserves to be treated fairly and equitably, and to have access to all the things non-disabled people have without a fight or a second thought. As you read this book, each story will more likely than not have something to do with The Chaeli Campaign, so you can appreciate how central this organisation is to my life. It's a complete privilege to have the opportunity to make a difference and to work with some incredible people who are equally driven by passion. This work is not just a job, it's an extension of our lives.

Chapter 2
For shits and giggles

I know that many people worry about this and wonder about it, so I'm going to share some stories with you about how I have handled bathroom-related drama in my life – and there are many. This may be the most inappropriate and gross chapter in the book, but hopefully it's also relatable at some level. I know it's a weird decision to tell people all about the most embarrassing moments of my life, but I don't really care. I hope that by talking about it, people who've been in similar situations won't feel as though they're alone in these experiences. To go with this, humour has always been a great coping mechanism for me, especially when I'm in shitty situations.

Are you ready?

There are so many things that remain unsaid when you live with a disability. Many people have questions that they don't find answers to because they're too scared to ask me, as they're not sure how I am going to respond. So many of these questions are about the private things nobody talks about, but we all have to do these things – pooping and peeing.

I've always had issues with incontinence and managing my colon. (Welcome to "sharing all of my business with Chaeli".) This has led to some pretty hectic experiences, but also some good realisations for me and those around me that we need to trust the people in our lives to support us in moments of crisis and embarrassment. What I love about all these colon-related dramas is that I never have these experiences on my own – I always share them with other people because I can't help myself. I've had some of the most open, honest conversations with my friends about how my body works (or doesn't) and it's led to better relationships and a lot less stress. I'd prefer not to have experiences like these, but they are experiences shared, and these are always good stories when you're reminiscing around a fire with a drink or two ... or when you write a book.

Most of my stories relating to this have happened in awkwardly public spaces and we've managed to find the funny side of the situation ... most of the time. Well, if not initially then definitely after the fact.

I've developed some code words for when I'm having a body crisis. Only a few people have been privy to this code prior to now, dear reader. So, if you already know these you can consider yourself inside the circle of trust. I definitely recommend designing a crisis code for yourself because it enables fast action with minimal communication requirements.

Chaeli's Crisis Code Starter Kit:

Chaeli's code	Meaning
"I'm having an issue"	This is used when the body is in an unreliable or critical state, on the brink of disaster. If these words are expressed, find Imodium and start looking for solutions, preferably a bathroom in the immediate vicinity. Hurry.
"We have a situation"	This is used when the first code is futile. It's too late. Shit has happened. Source a location for triage and commence containment strategies. Don't say "It's okay" right now. Tears will be shed if the situation is not handled swiftly.
"I'm having a moment"	This is about prevention and will generally be used in sporting contexts where meltdowns are highly possible. It can be used when things are emotionally and physically overwhelming. I will be having conversations with myself to prevent full meltdown mode and crying may occur. No action is required. If spontaneous sobbing starts, refer to the first code.

BODY REBELLION IN PUBLIC PLACES

When I thought about writing this chapter there was one story that immediately sprang to mind. One time, my body let me down on an aeroplane. (This has happened more than once, but this particular time was extra memorable/traumatic.)

Let me set the scene. We had been in Johannesburg for work – I can't remember exactly why we were there, but this is not the point of this story – and Mom was with me. I think I was about 19 years old. At this age, a person usually has control over their bodily functions, but alas, welcome to the unpredictability of disability. You must know that when we travel, we usually have 700 things with us in case of any eventuality. I'm disabled; I have a lot of (non-metaphorical) baggage. For some reason, on this day we decided that we were going to trust my body and believe that nothing was going to happen. So, we checked in all of the bags we had, including the emergency "everything" bag, because nothing bad was going to happen. I don't want to say rookie error because we were already 19 years in, but...

Rookie error.

Everything was going according to plan and I was feeling perfectly fine. We boarded the plane with the help of the passenger aid unit, which is a mechanical hoist used to lift wheelchair users and anyone who struggles to walk and needs assistance into an aeroplane. I remember I was in row 11 and I was sitting in the middle seat. This would not normally be an issue, but it's also a little weird because airlines have policies relating to disabled people and generally if you're an assisted passenger you either sit in the front rows or the back rows, but not this time. We paid no mind to this, as everything was super chilled. Until it wasn't...

All passengers had boarded the plane and we were getting ready to take off on the two-and-a-half-hour flight home. Little did we know that my body had other plans. Just as the crew were about to close all the doors, I realised we were about to encounter a serious body rebellion moment. I don't think I had eaten anything hectic to make my stomach unhappy – all I knew at that point was that my colon was making a power play. I looked at Mom and I think she instantly saw the panic in my eyes, and I said in the calmest way possible (read: not calm at all): "Mom, I need the bathroom."

It was probably the worst thing I could have uttered. I think these words have instilled fear in my family and friends more times than I (or they) care to remember. These incidents always seem to happen at the most inopportune moments.

Mom sprang into action, grabbing me and carrying me to the closest bathroom, which was behind us. I knew as soon as she picked me up that it was going to be a shit show. Any other day we would not be stressing, but on this day, we are entirely unprepared for this because all of our emergency supplies – extra clothes, towels, wet wipes, dignity – are chilling in the hold of the plane. So helpful.

Just to give you a better picture, Mom has a very particular way of carrying me over longish distances (actually, any distance, it's just her way). It's apparently the most energy-efficient method and takes things like momentum into consideration. Very scientific. She'll hold me with one arm under my right arm and then her other hand has me under my left leg, and then she will essentially throw me with the requisite energy and speed to ensure that I reach my intended seating destination. Nobody else has ever even attempted to carry me this way. If we have to move while in this position, we just use all our collective willpower to try not to collapse. I'm generally not at all helpful at times like this because I think it's funny, so I just get hysterical with laughter and it makes Mom mad because I get heavy. (I'm told that when I laugh, I triple my body weight.) This time, though, I wasn't laughing. It wasn't funny.

We reach the bathroom, and anyone who has ever been on a plane before will tell you that those bathroom doors are the most impossible things to work with and to keep open. Never mind the other obstacle, namely the width of the aisle, to reach the bathroom. It's a very small space at the best of times, and even more so when you're having a body malfunction. Definitely less than ideal for accessibility purposes. On longer flights there are bigger bathrooms (I think it's a few extra centimetres, but you can feel the difference), but not on domestic planes, and let's not pretend that we had any time to be picky about our ablution options. Anyway, we wrestle all of my limbs into the concertina bathroom door and fit both of our bodies into that tiny space.

Now that we are safely inside the bathroom, we can begin addressing the problem. I know that we are those "there are no problems, just solutions" people, but we really need to stop saying that in every situation. This was a problem.

Shit hit the fan in a big way. It was everywhere.

We have *nothing* with us to clean up or for me to change into, so right now we have no plan. While Mom starts removing pieces of clothing (mine and hers) as carefully as possible, I realise the extent of the issue and start panicking properly about the very minimal solutions we have at our disposal. Now I'm crying. Mom has the strategy of trying to make me laugh when I'm crying in an intense situation such as this. It really annoys me in the moment because to me it's clearly not a laughing matter when there is poop on the walls.

It's funny now ... seven years later. This story gets way more hectic and ridiculous. Hold on to your seats.

Mom devises a plan that I am 100% not on board with. She suggests that the only thing to do is remove all of my affected clothing, throw it away and wrap me in a blanket... In this moment, she thought I was just being difficult, and couldn't believe that her 19-year-old daughter didn't want to sit next to strangers basically naked. I mean, we had no options, right? Nope. There are always options if *that's* the only option. So, we're arguing about alternatives and there's a polite but assertive knock on the bathroom door. It's the flight attendant asking for a status update because at this point we have already delayed the flight by 25 minutes. I don't think we needed to explain the full situation – she pretty much understood what was happening as soon as we opened the door and she witnessed the explosion. We did actually need to involve her because we didn't have anything to put back on my body, so Mom conveyed the key information because I was no help.

She leaves. We continue with the cleanup in aisle two. She returns with supplies. Flight attendants are special people. They deal with so many disgusting situations from passengers, with a smile. I see and appreciate you. She comes back with her emergency kit (the irony is not lost on me), which contains a panty liner and a pair of panties. I still have no pants to wear, but not to worry, she has made a plan. Her colleague had an extra pair of tracksuit pants in his bag and has given them to us.

While we are dealing with the immediate crisis, the flight attendants organise to move us to the last row, closest to the bathroom. Just in case the madness strikes again.

I'm now relatively clean, wearing someone else's panties and an unknown man's pants. If that's not a low point, I don't know what is.

We have to find the emotional strength to open the door to return to the cabin where people have been waiting for 45 minutes for us to sort me out. Mom puts me in my newly designated seat in the back of the plane and I'm trying to become invisible to hide in plain sight because seriously, how could my body do this to me? I was unsuccessful.

I'm hoping that the plane just takes off and nobody makes any mention of what has just happened, but obviously things are never that simple in our lives. And obviously every member of the crew knows exactly what's going on (I'm wearing their clothes, I mean really). Before takeoff the pilot comes over the intercom and apologises to all the passengers for the delay, saying there was a problem with offloading some baggage.

And the award for understatement of the century goes to...

I'm sitting in my seat, refusing any food offered to me, avoiding eye contact with any human being, including Mom. The plane takes off and we're finally on our way home to Cape Town. Thank you. We can now put this horrid experience behind us. Again, nope.

Mom goes back to the bathroom to do some damage control. The flight attendant tells Mom that she doesn't have to do that, as we are their customers. I think they just wanted us to remain seated to avoid any more drama, but we'll accept it as good customer service too. There are some interesting things we learnt about how planes function in this whole series of events, though. Mom proceeds to attempt to mask the evidence and sprays deodorant. Seems logical. Turns out smoke detectors in plane bathrooms respond to deodorant too. I just close my eyes and act as though I have no idea why the alarm is going crazy. Mom is stressing now, and the exasperated flight attendant returns once again to these highly problematic passengers (that's us, if you were unsure) to see what the hell is happening now. Mom explains what she did and asks them if they can turn off the alarm because it's literally going off at full volume throughout the entire plane. Turns out you can't turn off a smoke alarm on a plane – you have to wait for the smoke to dissipate sufficiently and it will turn off on its own. So that's great.

In my opinion, anything that goes off automatically should also have a manual override function.

When we landed in Cape Town, it felt as though that was the longest flight I had ever been on in my entire life, even though it was only two-and-a-half hours. It always takes a while to get off planes when you're a wheelchair user because you wait until everybody else is off before the passenger aid unit comes to take you off. This was one of the times I was not so excited to be the last person to leave the plane, mostly because I really didn't want to meet up with the cleaning staff and witness their introduction to what we had done to the bathroom.

If you were on this plane … apologies. More so if you were anywhere near us. It was truly the most traumatic bathroom experience I've had in my life. Mom feels the same way.

I think there are some good lessons in this, though. First and foremost, try your best not to poop on planes. Second, never think that nothing will go wrong because there is always the potential for things to go somewhere you don't want them to go. It is better to be overly prepared for your body to be completely unreasonable and to leave you in the shit. So, always take everything with you and keep it close by – you never know when you're going to need it. And hey, maybe someone else has a body malfunction and you can pay it forward and help them out of a crisis.

When we eventually got to the parking lot where Dad was waiting for us, we got into the car and the first thing he said was, "Hi! Why was your plane delayed for so long?"

THE WEE HOURS

The second most memorable, and also preferably forgotten, airport extravaganza was an international one, so that was fun. It's great to know that your body doesn't care where in the world you are, it just does what it wants, when it wants.

It was 2018 and I was in Los Angeles to launch Chaeli Foundation USA. The trip was successful and we were really happy with how everything turned out. We were also excited to be in the US at that time because it was the midterm elections, and it was interesting to see how things worked in another country. This was not why we were there, but it was a cool bonus, nevertheless.

Vicki Graf, a professor at Loyola Marymount University in LA, is a good friend of ours. We met her at an inclusion conference a few years ago and have worked together on a few things for The Chaeli Campaign over the years. She is a professor of inclusive education and is an incredible networker; she's always willing to connect us with people who can assist us and collaborate. She now serves on the board of Chaeli Foundation USA and is a wonderful supporter of our work. We met up with Vicki at Loyola Marymount University and spent the day there because Dr Sofia Vergara, a lecturer in the Education Department, had invited us to chat to some of the students. Sofia is epic and also happens to have CP. Before heading to the airport we got some coffee and I waited in the queue with my American friend Jameson (we met at the 2012 World Summit of Nobel Peace Laureates in Chicago when I was awarded the Medal for Social Activism) to cast his vote for the midterms, while we waited for our transport to arrive. Contrary to popular belief, there are effective alternative options for disabled people to get to places, apart from parents with big-ass vehicles. This will not be confirmed in this particular example, because what came to our rescue? A parent with a big-ass vehicle. But the point stands.

[TANGENT]
In South Africa, I often use Uber to get around, but we don't have the Wheelchair Accessible Vehicle (WAV) option yet, like in the US. (Maybe it's coming... I'm holding thumbs.) So instead, we ordered the XL option, which is usually big enough to put my wheelchair in the back, and we put me in the front seat. I just have to make sure there's a person to put me into the

car and take me out of the car when I get to my desired destination (if I'm going on my own). This works pretty well, but because we were in the US and the WAV option exists, we figured we should give it a try. Initially, I didn't know we could do this, so the first time I ordered an XL because that's what we're used to. I also didn't know that you can't pay for your ride in cash, so when I got the credit card withdrawal message from my bank for almost R900 for a single trip (the exchange rate sucked), I almost cried. Lesson learnt. Thanks, life.

After a relatively unsuccessful string of Uber rides with crazily long waiting times (up to 45 minutes for the WAV options; drivers arriving and refusing to pick us up because of my wheelchair with the non-WAV options) I complained and we sorted this out when we got home. They were very helpful and solution-oriented.
[TANGENT OVER]

Throughout this trip we learnt that sometimes it's good to stick with what you know. This became clear as we attempted to get ourselves and our luggage back to LAX so that we could make our way home. The WAV Uber estimated arrival time kept changing – from 20 minutes, to 45 minutes, to 15 minutes. All this while our boarding time remained the same. So we went from having plenty of time to get to the airport to not being sure we would make it in time to check in in time. We were stressed. Sofia's dad has a wheelchair-accessible car and they offered to give us a lift to the airport before they went home. Amazing. Mom and I breathed a sigh of relief.

If you're wondering what this story is doing in this particular chapter, here it is. I think it's pretty fair to say that I suffer from FOMO, and as a result, I regularly ignore my body signals.

Earlier on in the day, before my presentation, I had already had a close call in the bathroom, but we handled it relatively well with minimal stress. However, because I now have my Mitrofanoff (this is a stoma for catheterisation, using my appendix – more on this later) we don't carry as many emergency supplies as we used to. I didn't have extra panty liners (we say "panty liners", avoiding infantilisation – it's the preferred term for me), so I had to just wear panties. Not a crisis in itself, but it increased my stress levels and bladder awareness because even though I have more control now, sometimes accidents happen and leaking can still occur.

Risky.

We were running late and there wasn't enough time to go to the bathroom before my talk. I figured I could just harness enough brainpower to keep my bladder in line. I forgot that my body doesn't always like listening to me. So midway through my talk, I leaked. It wasn't the biggest deal because I was sitting down and I had my table on, so nobody would notice if my pants were a bit wet. I've been thankful for this weird disability perk many times in my life. I was also focused on being professional, so my focus had migrated away from controlling my bladder.

At that stage my bladder could hold for two hours or so, and I forgot to set my internal reminder. I'm pretty good at not bringing attention to my body crises while they're happening in inappropriate places, so nobody was aware of the situation. I may have initially underestimated the magnitude of the issue. When I eventually checked the "water line" (five hours later) it was so far past okay that I was nervous about leaving a river behind me wherever I went. So I just sat very still until we had made a plan and Sofia's dad arrived to take us to the airport.

In the meantime Mom had repacked our suitcase – I can't remember why it needed repacking – and reinforced it with cable ties to keep our stuff safe and we were on our way to LAX. We figured that because I was already soaked, whatever we did in the car wouldn't make any difference. We would just sort it out when we got to the airport. Evidently, our suitcase was even safe from us. Given my previously mentioned body rebellions, we've proven that we actually don't always learn from past experiences. If we had, I would have had multiple outfit changes but nope. Not today. Again. All of my clothes are in our newly extra-secured suitcase. And do you think we have scissors with us to cut the cable ties? We did, but they were *inside* the cable-tied suitcase. So that was great. And where can you find a pair of scissors or anything sharp enough to cut through cable ties at an airport, you ask? Spoiler alert – you can't!

We solved this problem by "MacGyvering" a solution with whatever was in the car. It worked and we got the bag open.

We were now going to be late checking in but I was so desperate to find a bathroom so I could finally change my clothes and be dry again. We assumed that there would be bathrooms everywhere in the airport, but this was not the case. We thought we could go through to the security area and find a bathroom before going through the whole security process. Thinking about that decision now, I can understand why that wouldn't be an option. I can also see why the security people would think that we were acting suspiciously if we did that.

As soon as we unintentionally found ourselves in the actual security line and I realised that we had to go through security first, I tried to turn around and get out of the line like a puppy going to the vet for the first time and trying to leave the exam room. I think I made similar whimpering noises too. At the same time I was trying to keep as still as possible. My bladder had already exploded, I was wet all the way up to my boobs and I felt I was leaving rivers and puddles behind me. This did wonders for my self-esteem. A piece of my soul left my body just then; it probably decided to stay in the pee puddles... In my brain I was just pleading with the universe, "Please don't make me go there?"

I know how seriously the US takes security checks at airports, and when you're in a motorised wheelchair it's even more involved. I have no dignity or self-respect left, I'm in a state of anger, frustration, fear and utter embarrassment; I'm an adult and now I have a body that is acting like a toddler throwing a tantrum. I'm convinced everyone in the airport knows exactly what is happening (I recognise that in the moment I may have had an inflated sense of self-importance), so I'm avoiding eye contact because I'm not ready to confirm my suspicions. Mom and I are communicating silently about how we are going to broach the subject without causing a scene or having anyone think we were starting an international incident.

We get to the front of the line with our millions of bags, and I'm dying inside because I know they're about to start frisking me, and they're about to find out all my business when they feel the wetness all the way up my torso and down to my knees. The security woman grabs a pair of the blue gloves they use for searches and gazes vaguely in my direction, and my embarrassment barometer can't take it any more. I start crying, which I'll admit looks suspicious. Mom tries to explain to them why I'm crying and I think they understood, but they still insisted on doing their job. They heard the story and called their supervisor for her to decide how much of a risk I was. They still did the frisking. Granted, it was a less intense check than it usually is, even though when Mom tried to wipe the tears off my face they freaked out, saying, "Ma'am, you're not permitted to touch her during the search."

That seemed slightly extreme to me, given the situation, but okay, they're just doing their job... Every second of this search is taking a piece of my soul, indiscreetly making its new home in the puddle I am leaving on the floor. We make it through that experience, and I'm traumatised and embarrassed to my core. We leave security, soaking wet, completely undignified, to find a bathroom. Finally.

I take a few deep breaths and try not to think about what has happened. We pretend it didn't happen and continue with the original plan. I still remember it so clearly, so obviously that whole pretending thing wasn't too effective.

We still had a 16-hour trip back to South Africa to prepare for and live through. We reached the bathroom and sorted out my indwelling catheter for the long journey home. It felt like it took ages, because it did. For some reason, it took us almost 45 minutes to get everything done. Now we were even later for boarding, but I was unfazed at this point. Over it. If anyone was going to make a comment, I was ready to stare them down. Once we were on the plane and in our seats, everything went perfectly. However, it's important to note here that our standards or expectations of anything going well had been significantly lowered. Anything that wasn't a crisis became acceptable.

At least in the plane bathroom shit show it was just me and Mom; I didn't have to engage with anyone else until the situation was handled. Here, it was in a truly public place where there were literally hundreds of people near me and I had to admit in front of everyone there (even if it was just an internal conversation) that I had no control over my body. My disability won that day.

I have mixed feelings about airports. I try hard to go into them with as much optimism as I can, even after having had the above experiences. It's like my body recognises the airport and goes into a mode that's a mixture of anxiety, disbelief, overpreparation and denial. Apart from all my body drama, there is always stress about whether my wheelchair will arrive at our destination in one piece. That's a story for another day.

What could the lesson here be? It could be "just don't travel" – but there's no fun in that! I want to see the world, which means my body has to accompany me; it just needs to get its shit together so that I can go on more adventures.

Lesson learnt? I think the lesson I keep relearning through all of these body rebellions is how important dignity is, how fragile it is and how quickly it can fly out the window in any situation. Alongside dignity is its close relative, privacy...

JUST A MINUTE

I am never alone.

Privacy is not a thing in my life.

The nature of my disability dictates this. It wasn't and continues not to be a choice I have. By anyone's standards I am severely disabled, considering how much support I need and the list of stuff I need help with. It's a lot. I can be lot. I know this.

My argument is that I am less high-maintenance because I openly recognise and express how high-maintenance I am. When I speak to my friends about this they tell me that being high-maintenance is different from just having a lot of needs that need to be accommodated, but this is taking some time to sink into my psyche (internalised ableism, my old friend). I think it's the same as when you're dealing with a bully at school, and you claim and celebrate your big nose, your weirdly longer arm, your donkey laugh – it takes all the power of that "flaw" for mockery and it becomes more of a superpower. So, nobody can tell me I'm high-maintenance or I'm too much effort because I told you when you arrived at this party what you were getting yourself into. If you now have a problem, that's on you.

Sometimes I make myself tired with all of this stuff, so I get it. Sometimes I just want to be able to do things myself, but that's not the life I've been given. I know I need to find ways of doing things myself and being as independent as I can be. However, I also think that it's important to prioritise the things I have to do each day and decide which activities are worth spending my energy on. Brushing my teeth is not high on my energy-efficient activity list, so I get help with that. It's not lazy to choose to have help with certain things so that I can spend my time doing things that are more important to me. I'm not undermining my independence by asking for help. I'm saving the 20 minutes of energy (and frustration) it would take if I were to brush my own teeth, for other things.

Living with my disability teaches me that life is largely about compromise. You can't get everything you want, when you want it. I can't do a lot of physical things – getting out of bed, getting dressed, putting on makeup, eating peas … the list goes on – but that doesn't make me an incapable human being. I've decided that not being able to do these things doesn't need to occupy all of my brain space. So I have people around all the time. Just in case I need help with something. Even if they're not sitting next to me, they are still within shouting distance and always aware of me. This is not necessarily a negative thing because I am totally a people person and I would definitely get bored with my own company if I were on my own for too long.

My physical needs in terms of personal hygiene – bathing/showering, going to the bathroom, changing panty liners, fixing bras – are the same as other people's needs. I just need more assistance than others. I have to share intimate things with the people around me so that I can live my life. Privacy is a luxury and although everyone technically has the right to privacy, it's not a right that I can access. Everyone in my life knows all of my business, all of the time.

I could get really angry about this and rage against the unfairness of it all. But my anger or frustration is not going to change the fact that I still need help with all of these things. I think that being disabled my entire life has been a blessing in this regard because it wasn't something I had to get used to; it wasn't something that came suddenly and changed my understanding of myself. It's just always been here with me, and a part of me. I have always needed help. I dealt with it a long time ago. I think this may be a benefit when I'm an old woman – I won't be able to get grumpy with the world because I have lost my independence and need more help than I used to. I've needed this level of support for my entire existence, so no excuses there.

Privacy is just not something that exists in my life. I have to let that go. I will always have a roommate; I will never go backpacking solo through Thailand or travel anywhere on my own. I have to let that go. I'm never going to put myself on a toilet and wipe my own ass. I have to let that go.

I have to channel my energy towards the things I can control, otherwise I would be in a deep depression and not be able to function at all. As the saying goes, sometimes you have to lose the battle to win the war. I'm not upset that I need help or that my body has placed certain limitations on my life. It's hard when people don't recognise all of the smaller things that I have had to let go of in order to live a life that I believe is valuable and full, when those arguably small things (like helping me to eat) are made to be giant, seemingly insurmountable barriers. This can make positivity difficult.

I don't spend too much time worrying about these things, but sometimes I get tired of being positive and it hits home that it's actually really hard to be a disabled person, wherever you are. In these moments I'm not questioning why I'm disabled; it's more of a "Can I just have a minute?" thought. Not a minute to not be disabled, because that's not possible, but just a minute where somebody else can fully embrace and understand how hard it can be. A minute to breathe without the pressure of positivity – it's often a subconscious pressure I place on myself, as well as society doing that too. (I don't want to be your inspiration porn.)

I had an "aha" moment shortly after I got Eden. I was home for the weekend – I lived on campus for three years at university – and was working in my bedroom. Mom was out somewhere and Dad needed to go to the shop. He left and was gone for 20 minutes or so. I was safe; I had Eden with me. In those 20 minutes, I realised that that was the first time in my life I was alone, without a human being around me. It was weirdly freeing but also stressful. I was alone (not truly alone, but still, no people) and my mind went to a lot of places – freedom, and also a little bit of fear around "What if something happens?" but you can't make decisions dictated by what-ifs, and it was a powerful moment for me. I recognised how much I rely on people, not just in a physical sense but emotionally and psychologically too. I need people, and that's totally okay.

In my experience, private, intimate, embarrassing moments have always been shared experiences and shared memories. This can be good because relationships are built on making and sharing memories. (Bonding opportunities, right? Ha, but I don't always want these kinds of opportunities!) While this makes sense to me, I can also appreciate that because they've been shared with another person, that moment becomes part of that person's life story too. It's like how a secret is only a secret if you're the only one who knows about it. I don't have too many secrets. I appreciate, too, that privacy and not sharing because "it's none of your business" can also be contributing to the stigma around disability and all the things we don't talk about.

Some things we don't want to remember, and therefore agree never to speak of them again. I guess I'm breaking that agreement by putting this particular incident in a book like this, but I think I'll be forgiven because this story has some solid entertainment value.

Erin and I were in high school when Mom had to spend some time in hospital to have her gall bladder removed. I guess we could say Mom is generally my primary caregiver (this is also why she is in most of my stories...), so we made a plan. She was only going to be there for two days, so Erin would help me get ready for school and Dad would be on duty at night to turn me over and stuff. Seems simple enough, right?

I was in Grade 8 and with all the things that happen to your body when you're 14 years old (puberty is great), I wasn't comfortable with Dad helping with things like dressing me and changing me. I'm over that now. I'm now much less concerned about these types of things – I just explain what I need someone to do. We therefore decided it would be best if Erin helped me with anything requiring a lack of clothes. Pooping fits into that category.

We went to visit Mom in hospital and left just before 7pm. We had been home for not even 15 minutes when my body decided to take a moment and make a scene. We barely made it to the bathroom in time. Little did we know that this was the beginning of a war my body was waging on us.

After the fact, we joked that if my body had acted up a little earlier we would have been at the hospital and I could have had a bed right next to Mom. Clearly the story didn't go that way, and my sister and I ended up sharing a mutually unwanted life experience. Erin has always helped with a bunch of things so it wasn't new that she needed to help me now. This was one of the times I really wished I had more ability than I have, especially getting myself onto and off a toilet.

So, in a matter of hours it was literally a complete shit show. Erin and I had already had numerous arguments around trying to locate the exact moment or action that had led to this situation. What did you eat? Why aren't you more aware of and careful about what you put into your body? You have to tell me sooner, not after you've pooped! I would have, if my body had a solid warning system, but it doesn't really have one. It's kind of like when you buy kids' toys and they say "batteries not included". Tensions were high and frustrations were visible on both sides. I definitely didn't want to be living through that next-level gastro and Erin was completely over it after the fifth bathroom session of the evening.

I still don't know why my body and the universe chose to do the dirty on us like that. We can handle many things, but that was exhausting. Needing the bathroom every 10 minutes is quite excessive for anyone, regardless of disability. Eventually we decided that moving from the loo to my chair and back to the loo was a waste of energy. Erin had to be in the bathroom with me because I didn't have great core strength, balance or any of the skills required to keep myself on a toilet. Can you imagine if I had fallen off the toilet when there was so much going on? Erin's solution was to get a blanket and a pillow to set up a bed station in the bath, like she was preparing for a bomb to arrive. Not far from the truth, to be honest.

This went on for Mom's whole hospital stay. It was a long two days. Neither of us slept enough. If we had two hours of sleep between us, it was a lot. I wasn't keen on involving any more people than was absolutely necessary. Dad kept offering solutions, but we were so deep in the shit that we weren't really in a place to receive them with an open mind. Dad also had to go to work and Erin was handling the situation pretty well. We didn't go to school the next day because my body was still out of control and we also just needed to get some sleep. Not that that happened, but it was the intention. We determined after about 15 hours that it was much too cold to sit in the bathroom (bathrooms are not designed for long-term stays) and we changed strategies. Also contributing to this change was the fact that throughout the night my body had exploded so many times that I had no clean clothes to wear and all the towels in our house were dirty and unusable. It was a change born of necessity. We were also getting bored sitting in the bathroom and this led to a few arguments. Neither of us wanted to be in the situation, and although we couldn't change the circumstances of my intestines freaking out, we realised that we could control the environment in which that mess was taking place. So we decided that we needed a distraction... We took the commode that lives in the bathroom, moved it to the bedroom and watched series (switching between *Friends* and *The O.C.*) while my body did whatever it wanted. I don't know why we didn't think of this earlier, but we used this strategy until Mom got home, and we got a whole box of Imodium. I don't remember why we didn't have Imodium at the beginning of this debacle, but I have a feeling that we tried using it and it did nothing for me at that stage.

Sometimes you can't stop your body from doing something, so you have to make a plan and reach a compromise. You find a plan where you can do what you want and where your body can do whatever it needs to do. Everybody wins.

Ultimately, I've reached a point where I'm no longer embarrassed (to the core of my being) when these body rebellions happen. When that point is reached, I kind of put it down to a "disability moment" and make a plan to move forward. Generally, though, a few tears are shed in the process.

I'm happy that I've had this realisation because I can translate it into other areas of my life too. Example? The time Eden got explosive diarrhoea on campus...

Eden had convinced me to take her outside to go "busy-busy", but I had no idea of the magnitude of my dog's intestinal struggles that day. I had only had her for a few months, so I wasn't used to looking at everything as potential hazards; I hadn't yet mastered my "mom eyes". Eden had sniffed out and found some old chicken on the ground, and before I knew it she had consumed it, in typical Labrador style. I'm pretty sure she regretted that decision shortly thereafter because she has never again eaten anything she's found on the campus grounds.

We made it outside to a patch of grass just in time. (I tried to find a spot somewhere where nobody sits or eats or does anything.) Eden exploded and the look of pure embarrassment and shock on her face when she gazed up at me is something I will never forget. When she was done, she wanted to move away from the scene as fast as possible. I pretended that nothing had happened, and headed off with her to my next lecture, but I quickly realised we were not going to make it to that lecture – or any other lectures for the remainder of that day.

Eden could not even walk five steps without stopping to poop or just leaking everywhere while she walked. I wasn't as embarrassed as I thought I'd be, but I don't think I've ever seen Eden with so little self-respect. (I can relate.) I couldn't spend the whole day underneath a tree with her because I had to finish some assignments that were due the next day. I called Mom to come and fetch her so that she could be comfortably sick at home, free from judgement. I was living on campus during my undergraduate degree, so Mom took Eden back to my residence to be with my personal-care assistant until she felt better (and until she stopped pooping). "Disability moment" status extends to Eden too, since she is an extension of me.

We took Eden to the vet because this situation seemed to be never-ending and she was given the canine equivalent of Imodium. (Mom calls it "anti-poop".) She stayed at home for a few days until the risk subsided and she could get her energy back. I noticed in this time that my friends had become much more concerned about Eden's wellbeing than mine. Apparently, when I wasn't on campus they'd assume I was away doing something cool for The Chaeli Campaign, which was probably a fair assumption. But Eden always accompanies me wherever I go, so her absence was noticed. I also found out in these few days that one of my lecturers was much fonder of Eden than she was of me. I had had my suspicions, but her concern for Eden confirmed it. I tried my best to be polite in my explanation of her absence (because, you know, that elusive thing called dignity), but everyone wanted all the details until I tried every polite version of "She's shitting everywhere!"

It seems that I'm so prone to oversharing information that when I try not to, the people around me think there's something wrong. So, I guess I'll keep sharing.

SHARING IS CARING

I have unavoidable support needs – like help in bathrooms – in order for me to live my life. I don't want my needs to limit how I live. I want my needs to be recognised as something to accommodate and plan around, and then we can get on with whatever epic thing we're doing that day. Disability often requires compromise, we've discussed this (it's not automatically negative to compromise) and one way this has manifested for me is that my physical support needs have meant I need to have more intimate relationships with the people around me.

Sharing my needs and being open, honest and vulnerable fits with my personality, but it's not everyone's first choice. That's okay. Some prefer not to share all the details of their disability. Each person has to decide what they're comfortable with sharing – and that should be respected. As you've seen from the stories I've shared here, there are many instances where disability is not the sexiest of experiences. The key thing to remember is that just because we have to deal with some unsexy things doesn't mean our self-worth or self-esteem should be dictated by these moments. I've chosen to let people into my life and be part of the journey so that we can share the responsibility of finding solutions. Making this choice, I've been able to expand my life in beautiful (sometimes momentarily embarrassing) ways because I've grown my circle of trusted humans. So much of my brain space is taken up by crises and preparing for said crises – it's nice to be able to share that with other people and not be the one who has to make all the plans.

This level of honesty and openness is also a coping mechanism (some may say it's more of a test) to see who can deal with all my disability drama, and let's be honest, there is a fair amount of disability drama over here. Putting it all out there is one way for me to own my issues and my story. If we can talk about uncomfortable things (and still remember dignity and respect) it gets easier to connect on other important stuff.

I have a strange balancing act in which I expect people to be accommodating and to support my needs, but I'm also 100% ready for people not to be able to do that. Internalised ableism like this is hard to root out, but I'm recognising it more now so I can work on dismantling it from the inside out. That being said, we haven't yet overcome ableism, so discomfort is still an expected response. If people are okay with all the baggage and extra support I need, then welcome to the inner circle. Let's go on some adventures and make memories!

TRUST MATTERS

When you don't have privacy and need help with everyday tasks, you have to trust people. I need to trust people not only with my physical needs but also on an emotional level. It's hard to do this because there's always a possibility that sharing will be met with rejection, misunderstanding and a whole array of negative emotions. That's why it's important to me to have a strong sense of security with my trusted circle because if it's solid, I have a buffer of support when negativity rears its head (which is pretty regularly). Sharing private, intimate experiences (like pooping in front of someone) takes any relationship to the next level, and there's a deeper understanding of each other. It has a humanising effect too, because everybody has to use a bathroom – the only difference is the methods people use.

It's more difficult for me to trust people with information. Sharing the practicalities of dealing with my disability is matter-of-fact and can be treated that way. However, the bigger deal for me is dealing with the emotional impact of those practicalities. Trusting the people around me to hold space for that aspect of my life with respect and dignity, and allowing space for those needs to be valid is something I've had to work hard for. I don't always accept and trust that the support I receive is genuine. I'm grateful to be able to talk through these feelings with my friends and family, and debunk this belief for myself. I think this particular suitcase of baggage arises from high-school experiences. I'll go into this in more detail in a later chapter...

I believe that trust has its foundations in control. If you don't have control, then you have to have trust, and if you build trust, then you don't have to worry so much about having control.

Trusting the people in my immediate circle and being brave when it comes to expanding the circle helps me have more trust in strangers. I know, I know ... stranger danger and all that. Given my above dilemma of struggling to trust people's intentions, the irony is that as a disabled person I have to have *some* level of trust with strangers to get things done (simple things like opening doors or getting a cup of coffee).

My wheelchair is an extension of myself, and without it, my entire personality apparently changes. I can see why people say this. Having independence and agency changes everything. When I'm not in control of my wheelchair, for instance when I get into an Uber or we're travelling somewhere and my wheelchair has to go in a boot or into the hold of a plane, I have to relinquish control and trust that the people working with my wheelchair will respect it as the empowerment tool that it is. If they don't and my chair gets damaged and I can't use it, prepare for a *scene*! When required, I don't make a scene, I make a whole movie.

I travel a lot, all over the place. It's pretty much always for advocacy work; we don't really travel for leisure or go on holiday ever. There is always an element of activism whenever we go anywhere. Even just getting to our destination can be an adventure! Usually my go-to travel partner is Mom, but in the last few years I have started travelling with other people.

Life tends to offer growth opportunities out of necessity. Let me tell you a story...

I was awarded the Peace Summit Medal for Social Activism at the World Summit of Nobel Peace Laureates in 2012, and we have been involved in and attended this summit ever since. It is a remarkable event to be part of – a collection of people (including some legendary Nobel laureates we're able to engage and connect with) committed to making the world a better place. I always leave feeling so motivated that we do have the collective power to change the world. The summit is in a different country each time and in 2019 it took place in Mexico. We decided that it was a good idea to take a delegation to represent The Chaeli Campaign and Chaeli Foundation USA in that activist space. Mexico is a tricky place to get to from South Africa. It took many flights and long layovers but it was totally worth it. It was amazing!

[TANGENT]
It took us 32 hours (ridiculous) to get to Mexico and I was so tired when we got there. By the time we landed in Mérida I was sufficiently over travelling, as well as over my friend, Fanelo, who had been my designated travel buddy for the duration of the trip. (Most of the time only one person is allowed to go with you, so for that trip it was Fanelo.) When we arrived at the hotel, we looked at each other and agreed that we needed some time apart. It took us only a few hours to recalibrate and we were back to making memories together.

And of course there had to be some drama on the plane, otherwise what kind of Chaeli story would this be? When we landed in Mérida I waited for the passenger assist people to take me out of the plane. They didn't speak a lot of English, which in itself is not an issue. It only became an issue when they thought I had core strength (usually I can sit up, but not after a marathon travel trip like we had just completed) and one of the assistants walked behind me, saw that I had my hand on my wheelchair and assumed I could hold myself up, and without communicating he proceeded to unclip all the straps on the aisle chair. (This is the wheelchair used to get me out of the plane. It's skinnier than a normal wheelchair, with tiny wheels so it can fit between the aisles easily.) I lost my balance and fell forward; I basically kissed the tarmac. Luckily I've learnt to put my arms up and kind of turn my body to protect my face (thanks to CrossFit training), so it wasn't as disastrous as the horrified airline staff thought it was. The assistants got a strong talking-to when their superior saw what happened. You can't treat a disabled person as though they have the same physical ability as a non-disabled passenger. If that were the case, I wouldn't require their services. I responded with hysterical (somewhat panicky) laughter and got some tar burn on my wrists, but no harm otherwise. Our whole South African delegation was there watching, stressed. When they saw I was laughing they knew everything was okay... We were just bleak that Chris, one of our ambassadors, stopped videoing a few seconds before I fell on my face. I could have gone viral!
[TANGENT OVER]

A couple of months before the World Summit, I had been invited to be a member of the Global Leadership Council of Generation Unlimited – a collective of public and private entities and individuals connecting education and training to the changing world and empowering young people to become productive and engaged citizens. My first meeting was in New York, a few days after the Summit ended. This wouldn't usually have been an issue because Mom would normally have come with me. However, our delegation had a few members who were schoolkids and Mom was their designated guardian for the trip. This meant that she couldn't accompany me to New York. Cue my friend Ash. Ash lives in London now, but we've been friends since university. She was also attending the World Summit with our delegation, so it made sense for us to go from Mexico to New York and start a new part of my adventures – travelling with friends!

What a vibe! The two of us believe we are absolutely hysterical, so we were guaranteed a good time. I also know that Ash would do anything for me, so that alleviated a lot of my stress. We usually have moments of realisation of what could go wrong when we're on our way to do something epic. Ironically, we only really thought about this when we were in the taxi on our way to the airport to catch our flight to New York (via Houston, Texas). We'd been friends for years, but the two of us had never been anywhere on our own, where Ash was 100% responsible for supporting my needs. We found a good balance between her taking on the role of personal-care assistant and just being my friend. Ash was judged harshly as being a grossly unprofessional assistant when she was taking embarrassing pictures of me sleeping during the flights. When she realised there were a few judgemental stares in her direction, she swiftly defended herself, saying, "We're friends first!"

We were in New York for four days and had our share of drama. We left our hotel in Mexico at 4am (neither of us was happy about this) and when boarding the plane Ash made it very clear to the passenger assist people that I had no balance, as she had been warned about my earlier face plant. The first time Ash had to help me was on the flight from Houston to New York, when my catheter blocked. I use indwelling catheters when travelling long distances because it means we have less to worry about.

So, we hustled ourselves into the bathroom (again, battling those stupid tiny plane bathroom doors). We were in there for a while ... struggling slightly, figuring out the physics of keeping me on a toilet while removing my shoes and pants and inserting a new catheter. This is easier than it sounds because of my Mitrofanoff. We had confidence in our abilities right up until the plane started experiencing severe turbulence. In the end, Ash found herself sitting on the floor trying to put my shoes on while I tried to activate every muscle responsible for balance to make sure I didn't end up on the floor with her. When we got back to our seats it was time to order snacks and drinks. The flight attendant arrived at our row and told us not to worry about paying for the snacks because we had been having a rough morning so far and we had earned our snacks. Clearly our bathroom experience that morning seemed more traumatic to others than we felt it was. The rest of the flight was problem-free. We made friends with the man sitting next to us and had a great chat. We knew he was cool because he offered to help get me into my seat. It's at times like this that I know I'm my mother's child. I'm never one to give up an opportunity to connect with people and learn about them.

We had minor challenges in Texas: a slight catheter dilemma (hence our extended aeroplane bathroom stay), being in the wrong terminal and having to take a *train* to the correct terminal, and having to hurtle past (I'm not exaggerating) 45 other gates to get to our boarding gate, where an incredibly grumpy woman was waiting who referred to me as "the wheelchair". We have since realised that 45-minute layovers are definitely not for me. We felt confident that the rest of our trip would be relatively problem-free (within reason, of course), but that feeling only lasted for the duration of the flight because upon arriving in New York we discovered that my suitcase had not made it onto the plane and was still in Texas. Bags that belong to disabled passengers are apparently subject to more screening and checking, which takes longer than usual bag checks. I wouldn't have as much of an issue with this if my bag arrives when I do, but it doesn't seem logical to me for disabled people's items to be heavily scrutinised and then not prioritised when suitcases are loaded – there are important things in our bags like medication, medical devices and products (in my case catheters) that we need in order to function.

Luckily, when we landed in Texas I'd asked Ash to take extra catheters out of my suitcase just in case. Seems like we had some divine intervention there. So, bagless, we headed to the hotel, which was a whole adventure in itself, and arrived at about 9pm, ready to figure out how we would get my bag. Ash spent hours on the phone tracking down my suitcase, getting more and more frustrated and angrier with every phone call. By the time I went to bed at about midnight it hadn't arrived yet. The board meeting was scheduled for 7am. I needed to look professional, and I only had the activewear I had travelled in, plus whatever extra travel-standard clothes were in my backpack. Our hotel was a short walk from the meeting venue. The dilemma we now faced was that my wheelchair had been in the hold of two planes, and because it's cold in the hold, the wheelchair battery doesn't hold its charge like it usually does. And can you guess where my wheelchair charger was? In my suitcase! As it turned out, we needn't have worried because my bag was delivered to the hotel at 1am. We went to the board meeting and nobody knew we had solved 3 000 problems to reach that point.

After the meeting, everything else worked out and our time in New York was awesome. A few days in, Ash looked at me with a sudden realisation and said in a slightly panicky voice, "Chaels, what happens if you need the bathroom, like to poop?"

I assured her that it was fine because my body (read bowels) generally only works when we tell it to and that because there were no plans to tell it to do anything, I was confident that nothing would happen. And it didn't ... until our next flight. I don't know why my body feels the need to taunt and terrify us whenever we go near an airport...

We misjudged the amount of time it would take to get to the airport and didn't have time to change into comfy travel clothes, so we decided we would change once we had checked in for our flight. I had sort of been needing the bathroom since we left the hotel, but I wasn't sure. You know when you don't think it's urgent, but you also think your insides might explode any minute? That was the situation. But we didn't have time for such a crisis just then, so I ignored those feelings. After successfully checking in, I fought with an airport-safety guy about the protocol around motorised wheelchairs. He wanted to check it in like a bag and put me in a giant manual wheelchair to make it easier (for whom?). He gave Ash a look that said, "Can you manage your disabled person?" but she stood back, knowing I had the situation under control and he shouldn't have started this conversation. I just told him we weren't going to do that because I've travelled all over the world and we never do that; it's not my responsibility to make your job easier, dude. In the middle of this argument, when I was telling this man we had to go because we needed to go through security, I remembered that one of the perks of being a wheelchair user was about to backfire on us...

I'm always sitting and have a table on my wheelchair, which means that when putting clothes on, we only need to worry about what people can see. This means that pants are often an optional bonus. I was wearing a pair of tights and I had a longish fancy shirt that we had strategically placed so I was decent. It usually works perfectly. But now we realised that when you go through security they take off the table to do their frisking. I'm trying to present myself as a totally-in-control disabled person who should be taken seriously, and here I am roaming around an airport pants-less. Anyway, we found a bathroom so we could change me and find some pants before I completely embarrassed myself in front of a whole lot of people. This was also the moment when I realised my tummy felt dodgier than usual.

We were about to embark on a long-haul flight. We had a five-hour flight from New York to Amsterdam, a three-hour layover and then another 12-hour flight to Cape Town. I had pants on now, and an indwelling catheter, but we were running out of time for boarding, so weren't able to shorten the pipe of the catheter collection bag – these are always *so* long. (Also, as mentioned previously, you can't have scissors at an airport, even if it's for medical reasons.)

We had devised a system where only one of us was allowed to be externally stressed or panicked at a time, so if I was stressed at a particular moment, Ash had to be the one to hold her shit together, and vice versa.

I had successfully distracted myself with some defensive sleeping, and my body forgot about its bowel-purging urges. When we arrived in Amsterdam it woke up and I needed to get to a bathroom asap! This was a major test of my ability to control my internal organs because it usually takes a minimum of 20 minutes to get me off a plane and into my chair. Luckily for us, the airport staff at Schiphol were super organised and were ready when we landed. Ash was chatting to the flight attendants and ground staff and thanking them for being so helpful while I was trying to remain polite and telepathically communicate my increasingly urgent need for a bathroom. I popped in a request for directions to the closest accessible toilet and Ash was back in assistant mode.

We got me on a toilet with seconds to spare – we were already at the goose bumps stage, so it was a high stakes game – but I was super impressed with my ability not to poop everywhere (Chaeli 1 – CP 0). Once the initial stress of that situation had subsided, we continued the conversation we had started on the plane, before the passenger assist people arrived. It's amazing to me that I have friendships where we can push through such awkward interactions and we've normalised the fact that I need help.

It's definitely taken many years to reach the point I'm at now. I'm proud that I've been able to let go (mostly) of being embarrassed when my body makes a scene and also lets go.

You may have noticed I like being in control. I feel this is due, in equal parts, to my personality and my disability. I don't always have control over my body and what it does, so I like to be in control of the situations I find myself in. Now obviously, given all the stories above, this is not always possible, so it's important for me to have strategies and ready-made plans to help me overcome barriers and have adventures. I'd like to take this moment to mention that not every moment in my life has a crisis component, but I'm always ready for it. I'd argue that overwhelmingly we are not in control of what is happening in our lives, and so these strategies become all the more important. Pay attention to your feelings and take the time to develop strategies that work for you.

I don't always succeed in managing my emotions in stressful moments, and I'm getting better at recognising the things that trigger my anxiety. Friends and family are helpful in working through these moments and we have devised a plan that works well in my life. I encourage you to give it a try and to create your own variation if you find it at all helpful. It's called the three-minute rule and it's really simple. It goes like this:

Something intense happens (it can be anything); you're completely overwhelmed by whatever it is and you have an outburst of all the emotions (for me this manifests in extreme crying). With the three-minute rule, you allow yourself to feel those feelings as intensely as you need to. Then you recognise that you need some time to process everything that's happening, but you don't necessarily have time for a full reflection.

If you really do need more time, just a few more minutes to gather yourself, there is a way around this without negating the strategy. It's called a "Mycroft minute". Our family's interpretation of time passing can be slower than what is standard. This means that you have "extra" time, but it can still count as three minutes.

Crises can be imminent and ever-present. This is a pretty terrifying, anxiety-inducing headspace to live in for too long or too often. I believe it's important to give a crisis its moment, but we also need to be able to share the load of the drama and let people in. If I were going through all of this by myself, I don't think I'd be as positive about it. Sharing it and acknowledging how ridiculous my body and disability can be is how I manage to find the funny side ... eventually.

Chapter 3
Learning as we go

Education has always been important to my parents and this value has been instilled in Erin and me too. My educational journey has had so many ups and downs, and I have had to have a lot of resilience and perseverance to reach my academic goals. This is a difficult aspect of my life to put into words. Putting it all down on paper has been a struggle for me, so I hope you'll just bear with me here. I don't want this to be a blame game or any kind of pity party. It definitely wasn't all bad. I'm just sharing my experiences and their impact. I believe that life experiences (lived moments, not just time spent on Earth) bring expertise, and getting an education as a disabled person is a hardcore journey that has, for sure, given me some expertise. The route my family and I have taken is certainly not the easy option, but looking back I am grateful for the opportunities I've had and the lessons I've learnt, which I take with me wherever I go.

This journey has taken me all over the place. I started at an inclusive day mother (I was the only disabled kid there), moved to a special-needs school and then went to a mainstream school at the age of nine. I continued with mainstream high school and went on to university, where I have acquired a number of degrees. Sounds simple, right? It was anything but. There is so much to talk about, so much to share, so much to process. Each stage is distinct, with different challenges, many of them arising from attitudes towards my disability rather than my disability itself. We'll get to all those stories, but I just wanted to lay it out like this so that you can see that although this road is long, with many twists and turns, we make it out in the end. Stronger and more determined.

DISABILITY MAKES A DIFFERENCE

My world has always been pretty able-centric, which isn't necessarily a negative thing. I think disability can be very isolating a lot of the time, but it doesn't have to be. Having a circle of able-bodied people around me didn't automatically leave me feeling left out or misunderstood, or make me feel I was at a disadvantage. In my circle, whatever we did was just adapted when necessary to accommodate my disability. I have family and friends (who are also basically family) who have never treated me "less than" because I'm disabled. My existence has been framed for me to expect that those around me should see me as capable, and for me that is an unbelievable gift that I am constantly reminded of. I guess this has served as a sort of protective bubble to protect me against the way the rest of the world may (or does) see me, and it has given me something to fall back on that I know to be true, when things get hard.

When I started going to our day mom, Aunty Jenny (she's the best!), my sister and our lifelong friends were there with me, so I don't think it was as tough as it could have been. I was surrounded by people who knew I could do stuff and treated me that way. I didn't get special treatment in terms of having different rules apply to me. My needs were accommodated, but I had to eat my veggies just like everyone else. Aunty Jenny made sure of that! When I was a little terror to my sister, a note was sent home to my parents, as would have happened with any other impossible toddler.

[TANGENT]
My parents had some rules and boundaries that were drawn with clear, solid grey lines.

Example. When we were really young and I was just about able to sit up on my own without falling over immediately (this phase lasted until I was about 20 years old – just a little longer than usual!), I was allowed to bite my sister, but it was a major no-no for her to bite me. Let me explain why. Erin is 15 months older than me. Older siblings always find ways to bother, annoy and tease their younger siblings. This was (and still is) no different for us just because I have a disability. She just found different ways to do this. Don't worry, I wasn't defenseless... I found my own tools for retaliation: my teeth.

This particular double standard was all about logic, practicality and just enough frustration to make it okay. The rule was: if you are going to irritate and taunt your little sister, do it at a distance. If she was close enough for me to sink my teeth into her, I was allowed to do so because she wasn't playing smart in her taunting techniques. Now, this is not a one-sided rule because we each had an opportunity to experience some level of enjoyment, depending on the outcome. My sister had the upper hand when she found the perfect distance to irritate me without risking injury, and I was winning when she had a lapse in judgement and came close to test our duelling skills, and I got the sweet taste of revenge and could use the spasticity in my jaw to my advantage.

Just to be clear, we don't do this any more. We stopped when I was about six years old, probably because it's not polite to bite people when you're at school. Our fighting/arguing has taken a more sophisticated turn now that we are older. Another point to clarify here is that our relationship is solid. Siblings get under each other's skin and that's just the way it is, so why should we be denied these little arguments and skirmishes? If I irritate my sister, she moans, and I do the same when she annoys me. We don't want to be held to a higher standard – that pedestal is too high.
[TANGENT OVER]

When the time came, it was a struggle to find preschools that would accept me. I've realised that this was the start of people defining me by my disability. It meant I was different, and different is often interpreted as being more difficult. I was fully included until I started my official schooling with preschool.

School became a much more complicated process when my parents started looking for a preschool because 20 or so years ago the world wasn't as open and accessible as it is today (which is still pretty closed). You would think that the perfect solution would have been for me to attend the same preschool as my sister, but it didn't work out that way. This is one of the reasons for starting an inclusive preschool and enrichment centre through The Chaeli Campaign. Here, parents can have peace of mind that their children's needs are being met, and siblings can learn together.

Preschools were hesitant to accept me primarily because I wasn't yet potty-trained (still working on this one), and they argued I would need more support than your typical toddler. I mean, technically they're not wrong. I kind of get it... It's daunting being asked to support a child with a disability and it's much easier to say no when something makes you nervous or doesn't fit into the prescribed, predetermined plan. At the same time, I'm not sure that's enough of a reason to say no. Maybe we give each other too much wiggle room when it comes to doing the hard stuff. I think doing something or not doing something because of fear is not a great basis for any decision. I'm still working on this strategy myself, though, so don't think I'm sitting here in judgement.

This is the reality for far too many children with disabilities and we have a long way to go before we reach a point of equitable access to education. I chose to make this topic the focus of my master's dissertation, so if you want to see a more academic approach to this issue, I'm sure you can find it somewhere. Right now, I'm not wearing my academic hat, I'm just wearing my "this is my life" hat.

So, I had to go somewhere else. Somewhere different from where my sister and friends went, where my physical needs would not be the barrier they were deemed in the mainstream space. A big challenge in finding a school was finding a place that would not only support my physical needs but would also stimulate learning and challenge my academic potential. Remember that disabilities and the way in which they need to be accommodated are unique, and it's problematic that the system tries to place disabled children in a single box. I'm getting "activisty" again. Sorry not sorry.

Anyway, I went to a special-needs school from the age of three until I was nine. This was a bit of a weird environment for me initially because I wasn't surrounded by many disabled people in my everyday life, but then I started school and all my peers were disabled in some way. Even though I ultimately left to go to a mainstream school, I think attending a special-needs school was a crucial part of my journey of accepting my disability. In society, you don't see disabled people everywhere you go. Obviously, some people have hidden disabilities and there's no way to determine just by looking at someone that they're not disabled. But when you're at a special-needs school, you know that everyone there has some sort of challenge because otherwise they wouldn't be there. To my three-year-old self it was cool to learn that everyone has issues, and you can't always see them, but there are ways to support those challenges.

When I think back on that time in my life, it was a positive and happy experience. I remember the widest hallways; wheelchairs, walkers, standing frames and tricycles everywhere, each with the name of its user; the therapy room, where you'd find the most dedicated and special therapists; the seamless accessibility; the helpfulness of the teacher's assistant, who was there in a second if you needed anything... So many positive memories. Having disability paraphernalia and assistive devices everywhere you looked (and actually using them) was normal. I rode my tricycle all over the place; I used my walker to get around, even if it took a while longer than it would to use a wheelchair or another mode of transport; I wore my splints (all of them) and I went for my therapy sessions (all of them). It wasn't weird that I did these things, or that I sometimes needed to do things differently. Our classes were always small, and I was always the most severely physically disabled kid in the class, at least as far as I can remember.

We are a family of big moves. We don't really do things slowly or in small increments. Make a decision and then execute. If you're going to do something, be like Nike and just do it!

The thing about big moments is that they don't always come with a warning sign or a welcome parade. Often, they're disguised in everyday, mundane activities that turn everything on its head and lead you on a path that you never expected. It was a Wednesday and I was dropped at home after Brownies. (Yes, I was a Brownie, and it was amazing.) After getting me out of the car, Mom started chatting to my friend Hannah's mom. Hannah went to school with me and we did Brownies together, so her mom sometimes gave me a lift home. I went into the house, not knowing that my life would change after a pavement chat. Mom still firmly believes that these can be the most important chats, and I tend to agree. The lesson here? Take the time to speak to people, as it could change everything.
This particular chat started with a comment about our schoolwork and the curriculum. During this conversation, Mom started thinking that maybe it was time to question what the best place was for me, and maybe it was time for something new. After a relatively long time standing on the pavement,

Mom and Dad had a fairly long discussion on the stoep. (Our stoep is where all our big decisions are made and our strategies are devised.)

I was then brought into the conversation for my thoughts. They asked me how I would feel about testing out the whole mainstream school thing. I was excited at the opportunities of this new experience and being challenged in a new way. The decision was made. I would be going to a mainstream school – the one where Mom taught. The time between making that decision and my starting at the new school was probably three days. It was a Wednesday, so I finished the week and started the following Monday.

I was so excited. I didn't have a motorised wheelchair yet, so on my first day, Mom took me to where we had to line up before assembly. It was a great day to start because my class was going on an outing that day, so it was a more chilled introduction, at least for the first day. We hadn't realised that because of the nature of the outing everyone was allowed to "Sometimes you have to shout to be heard." Many may construe this as something negative, but I didn't see it that way. I loved that my disability wasn't a reason to get everything I wanted. I had to learn, once again, that I had to use my voice. I had to back myself and be just as vocal as any of the other kids in my class. I think this has been one of the greatest lessons and it's one that I keep relearning at different stages of my life.

At the end of that school year our challenges were drastically reduced, as we no longer had to compete with two flights of stairs to get to my classroom. The rest of primary school (that's four whole years) was all on the ground floor!

Grade 4 was a big year, not just in an academic way but also in a life way. This was the year I got my motorised wheelchair and it was the beginning of The Chaeli Campaign. We had no idea of all the places it would take us, and that's the amazing thing about life. We make one decision and it leads to so many possibilities. I was nine years old, having opportunities to speak at different schools, to talk about what we had achieved and to encourage others to get involved. This stood me in good stead for future speaking engagements because when you've been doing something since before you've reached double digits it isn't that scary, and now I don't get nervous when I'm asked to speak in front of people. Winning.

We started The Chaeli Campaign in April that year. Seven weeks later I had my motorised wheelchair, and in August we formalised it as a non-profit organisation. See, here is another example of how we make decisions and act on them with a fair amount of (considered) speed. It feels like this was the year that a new life began. I don't remember what we did with our time before we had The Chaeli Campaign. Activism and advocacy became a bigger focus and I'm so grateful because I truly believe it is my life purpose. I've spent most of my life living out my purpose, and that's a special gift that I don't ever want to take for granted.

So, with all these things going on, I went to a number of events during school time. My family and I live by the philosophy that not all learning happens in a classroom. Having these opportunities and going into different communities for advocacy was teaching me life lessons that I would never be able to learn within the four walls of a school classroom. In my reality, most learning happens when we're not in a classroom – when we're just engaging with other people and figuring out how we can all work together in unique and beautiful ways.

wear civvies. (I don't remember where we went, I just remember there were birds involved.) I was in my uniform. Not a crisis; there wasn't enough time for me to get changed, so we just had to roll with it. I'm used to standing out (pun intended) and it was just another opportunity for that. On the bright side, being in my wheelchair meant that I wasn't running around getting super dirty anyway, so wearing my uniform that day became much less of a deal to me.

Being in a special-needs school was a good place for me to start, but now I needed something else that challenged me and my ability in new ways.

Many people underestimate how much we had to believe that it would work for me to go into mainstream schooling. And it's not just my immediate circle who had to have faith in this plan, it was the teachers too. I have had a few people in my life who have been undercover game-changers, and two such humans are both my Grade 3 teachers (at the special-needs school and my new mainstream school). If these women had been less supportive it could have been a very different situation and experience for me. Mrs Dobbie from my special-needs school was on board from the moment my parents informed the school that I would be leaving. Mom went back to her every so often for a while and she admitted that she had never thought about mainstreaming me because of the extent and severity of my physical disability. Then, when I moved, as luck would have it, the only grade that had its classes upstairs was ... you guessed it, Grade 3. It wasn't a major obstacle for us because it was already October, so we only had to find a solution for a few months. Mrs Vink was my teacher during this time, and she definitely ran a tight ship. You always knew where you stood with her. She was one of the most important people in my early educational journey because she saw and believed in the possibility of my inclusion. We often don't recognise how important a role certain people have played until moments like this, when you write a book. Maybe we should all write our stories so we can remember those who have made things possible for us. If she had been negative and said no to me joining her class, I could have found myself on a very different trajectory. I'm so thankful that she saw the situation as she did. I think it turned out pretty well ... mostly.

Obviously, we had to make some plans and figure out a few things. For example, we needed to find someone who could be my facilitator at school, especially considering the whole upstairs classroom issue. I would no longer have access to therapies during my school day, so we had to find a physio I could go to after school. At that point it was decided that we would focus on physio and go from there. I was supposed to have a two-week trial, after which we would determine the way forward. Those two weeks felt like a long time, as we were in a kind of limbo. We needed to know how everyone was feeling because we still hadn't made plans, and we had to know whether it was a permanent plan.

The school was really great about making sure there were accessible routes to the places I needed to be – ramps were constructed within a couple of weeks. It just proves that something is possible if it is deemed important enough. And yes, those ramps were installed for me, but I couldn't take them with me when I moved on to high school, so those spaces will be accessible for whoever needs them in future. It was an investment in future inclusion. There were a few conditions for me to stay: I had to have a facilitator, and I couldn't come to school if my facilitator wasn't able to come in for whatever reason. These felt reasonable at the time, and having Mom teaching at the school eased concerns considerably and smoothed the transition process.

It was definitely quite a culture shock. It was very different to being in a special-needs school in pretty much every way. A couple of months after moving to the school I was asked what I liked about it. My reply was,

How things change

When I moved to a mainstream school, even though it was ultimately a good decision for my life, I had left a safe and supportive space where accommodating my disability – like having everything in place to do all of my therapies – was part of my school day. Suddenly, doing these things meant extra work for me. This made my disability so much more obvious because it now meant making additional plans.

I was in Grade 3 (so basically at the start of my mainstream school journey) when I refused to do bubble-blowing sessions while everyone else was doing recorder lessons. We then found creative alternatives to therapies, like singing lessons and joining the school choir. This was the start of me giving a lot more pushback with wearing splints and doing other therapeutic things. For instance, when I turned 12 I no longer wanted to ride my tricycle during break.

At a certain point in life, what people think starts to matter more. (Not that it should, but it does.) I didn't want to do different things from all the other kids, things that pointed out my disability so blatantly – more than my wheelchair did, at least in my mind. I didn't want to ride my bike at school any more because nobody else was allowed to ride bikes. I didn't want to be in my standing frame in class any more. (It was before the whole standing-desk trend.) I got really self-conscious about wearing my foot splints, so we made a pair that weren't as visible, as they fit inside my shoes. I eventually hated wearing my hand splints too because they were bulky and I felt like I looked like a lobster when they were on, and I was actually less functional wearing them. Thinking ahead, there was no chance anybody was going to get me to do any of these things when I got to high school. Then I would have been the smallest lobster in a big ocean with sharks, and I was not about to do that. Sometimes the social aspect of life is more important than the therapeutic benefits of an activity, especially when you are a teenager.

This was happening in about Grade 6, which is also the time that puberty was kicking in for me and my peers. I guess that could somewhat justify my increased resistance to everything we had always done. I felt there was a change in attitude towards me during this time, too. (I can't quite put my finger on it. It wasn't obviously negative, more like an undercurrent mood shift.)

There were a few moments and incidents that made me think this. I can think of two examples. When we were in Grade 7, there were no prefects because every Grade 7 was given a job. Some jobs were more intense or had more responsibility than others. I applied for Class Monitor roles (this entailed being with a particular class, making sure they were all in their line before school, after break and so on), but I didn't get any of the jobs I applied for. Instead, I was given a job that required minimal effort and responsibility. I don't believe there was any malice behind this decision, but I feel my disability did impact the decision. The second was the school play. These took place every two years and every pupil at the school was involved in some way. I don't know how this happened, but I was never assigned a part in the play. Clearly there was some kind of miscommunication, and I was also starting to investigate the whole "I'd rather be an invisible teenager" vibe, so I wasn't necessarily fazed by being left out. That was until Mom started asking me questions about the play and she eventually got that information out of me. I think there was an element of embarrassment that I had been left out and that I hadn't stuck up for myself or made a scene, demanding a part in the play. Ultimately, I was given a role because Mom stepped in and made sure of it. I ended up having a lot of fun with that, so I'm glad I didn't miss the opportunity. I'm still a little unsure of how that situation even occurred. Maybe it was a weird sort of life foreshadowing or something – a mini dose of what was to come.

[FLASHBACK]
I was in Grade 11, sitting in assembly, and we were watching a short film on cyberbullying. This was a random emotional trigger, as I've never experienced cyberbullying myself, but it did help me realise a few things about my own school experiences and the impact these have had on my life.
[FLASHBACK OVER]

High school was harder. Most of it was quite shitty, actually. Thinking back, I don't know how kids make it through high school. It's like a war zone and a jungle all rolled into one. At least that was my experience, but I'm prepared to bet some good money that I'm not alone in this.
I was excited to go to high school, meet new people, grow my circle and have a new environment. Just like a lot of things in my life, a fair amount of planning went into going to high school. It was suggested by our preferred school's management that we should submit my application a year early, so that they could make plans and get the school ready for me – at least the

physical accessibility – when I reached Grade 8, so we did that. I applied in my Grade 6 year. It was the closest high school to where we live, so that made sense too. The school was working with the Department of Education to negotiate funding for an elevator because it's a double-storey school. These negotiations were ultimately successful because money was allocated to get a lift installed before I got there. This was all a really great plan, in theory. (What is it they say about the best-laid plans?) In reality it didn't happen as smoothly as that.

I believe in giving people the benefit of the doubt and I'm always ready to make a plan if something is not working as planned or we have to navigate inaccessible spaces. For this to work, though, everyone involved should preferably be on the same page. Attitude (of everyone involved) is a crucial factor because if I'm the only one looking for solutions it's like running into a brick wall and it's just an uphill battle. Perhaps if I had been surrounded by more people with more positive outlooks, the less than ideal design of the school wouldn't have been the massive barrier it became.

[TANGENT]
When people talk about accessibility, many immediately think of ramps, lifts and the like. High school taught me that the existence of a ramp doesn't automatically mean you're in an empowering environment. It's more important to me to have people with open minds and positive attitudes around than having a perfectly physically accessible building. I can forgive a fair amount of physical inaccessibility if I have sufficiently positive minds around me. We can make a plan if need be. I've had to wait and fight for a long time to find people who have this in my life. This is not the part of the story where I tell you that everything gets better, because it actually got a lot harder for me before it got better. It took years to get better.
[TANGENT OVER]

An agreement was reached about putting in a lift before I arrived in high school, so that was exciting, but the lift was only installed at the end of my Grade 8 year – a full year after I started. I don't know what happened to the great strategy we spoke about earlier. My introductory year of high school wasn't particularly memorable for positives or negatives. It was hard to make friends, though. It felt like there was a short window of time you had in which to build friendships before the cliques were formed and solidified, and I sensed I may have missed that window.

I didn't feel particularly supported when it came to accommodating my disability needs at high school.

There are some ideas common in disability discussions that confuse people, like reasonable accommodation. We often get stuck on the idea that "everybody should be treated the same" and we can't see past this to reach equitable treatment. Another challenge in building common ground (in any context where inclusion is the goal) is how we understand the word "reasonable". Things that are perfectly reasonable to me are completely unreasonable to many others. It's also not a synonym for "unfair advantage" as a result of being disabled. This concept doesn't make sense to me. This has been an ongoing conversation in my life since I started at a mainstream school, and high school didn't change this.

A big deal that threw a new, unexpected spanner in the works happened at the start of my first high-school exam series. In the June of my Grade 8 year my facilitator left and started a new job. (Admittedly, the timing wasn't great, but this all worked out for the best eventually, and we're all good now. No hard feelings!) It turned out to be another blessing disguised as a crisis. It didn't feel much like a crisis to me at the time, but it was a pretty monumental wake-up call and forced us to re-evaluate our choices and reasoning behind those choices.

Mild panic ensued and multiple solutions were thrown into the ring. One suggestion was Mom coming with me every day. I wasn't excited about that, considering I was in high school, and high school can be filled with some of the most judgemental people (especially when you're an adolescent, surrounded by other adolescents, with hormones all over the place). Adding my mom to that equation would not have led to a desirable outcome for me. Mom did end up coming in with me that morning to explain the situation and also to negotiate with the deputy principal, who was in charge of the exam schedule/classroom allocation, because my class had been assigned an upstairs classroom for the entire exam series. This was a bit of an oversight on their part. My class was moved downstairs the next day and that made the rest of my exams much less stressful. It's funny to think that exam stress in my life generally had very little to do with actually writing the exams...

When we thought about it in more detail, I didn't actually need someone to be there with me 100% of the time. As it was, I was "flying solo" in my classes anyway because my academics didn't require any additional facilitation. All I needed help with was getting into my classes and getting set up with my books and stationery, and then I was good to go. So, when this "crisis" happened, we decided that I wouldn't have a facilitator at school, and we took the leap into this new unknown. It was empowering in a weird way, but not having a facilitator did take some getting used to. I had to make my own plans and be my own advocate in a way I hadn't needed to before. I don't think everyone in the school leadership team was happy with this decision, but it just didn't make sense any more, and having a facilitator was actually creating a barrier because I was seen as being someone else's job. This was a big hurdle because arriving at the school with a facilitator meant that that picture had solidified in people's minds, and asking or expecting them to now change that picture (and how they interacted with me) was a big thing and humans are not always great when it comes to adapting to change.

The best thing was when my timetable worked out in my favour and I had two, sometimes three, lessons downstairs at the start of the day. It meant I didn't have to hustle and fight to get into a classroom for a few hours. This didn't happen often, though – maybe once every two weeks.

When I started going to school without a facilitator it wasn't a massive shock to my system because I was already holding my own in a classroom. I *was* shocked, though, by how much resistance there was when I asked people to help me get into a classroom. Not too many people were keen to get involved. My homeroom teacher and a few other teachers were super helpful and supportive – carrying me up and down the stairs and getting me to the classes that were upstairs or less accessible – and they got some of the boys in my class to help them too. These teachers went above and beyond what was expected by the school to ensure that I had an easier time during the school day, and I truly appreciate their effort and care. The problem is that I wasn't spending most of the school day with these teachers.

At this stage there was still no lift. I had a manual wheelchair that we used when I had class upstairs because it was lighter and easier to carry. Carrying 60kg (wheelchair and me) up and down stairs every 45 minutes was not a workable solution. This didn't do great things for my sense of independence, but sometimes you don't have a lot of choice. This wouldn't have been as much of an issue if the lift had been installed as promised, but alas...

At the end of that year, I was hopeful. I remember thinking that Grade 9 was going to be easier because there would be a lift, and I wouldn't have to stress about how I was going to get to my upstairs classes. However, I didn't realise that puberty and all that comes with it would accompany us all to Grade 9, and this complicated life more than expected because navigating high-school drama and hectic hormones at the same time is a lot to deal with. That positive feeling that I had had before swiftly dissipated when I arrived at school on the first day of the new school year only to find that although the lift had been installed, it wasn't functional. I was told that there were mechanical challenges. (It was a case of scheduling the mechanic to come and make it functional.) Eventually everything was sorted out and the lift worked. It could only be used four months into my Grade 9 year. It sat there, taunting me. A subtle, everyday reminder of where my needs were placed on the list of priorities for the school.

I think this was when I really started disliking and not wanting to go to school. The design of the school building was problematic for any potential wheelchair users who were either attending or visiting the school. This is because even though the lift was now working, getting around was still a mission for me, if not necessarily physically, then definitely emotionally.

The lift would get me to the first floor, but there were sublevels (accessed via three steps), which meant that when I got upstairs, I still needed help to get up those steps to most of the classrooms. There were only four or five classrooms that I could access on my own and I didn't have classes in any of these, except in Grade 10. The class opposite the lift was Business Studies (which was one of my electives), so that was fairly simple. The design of the lift was as follows: it was open on one side with three sides closed and it had a manual safety arm across the front to stop anyone from falling off. I couldn't lift this arm on my own, so I needed somebody to help me lift it at both levels anyway. The lift worked with a remote; I think there were three of these. It didn't have buttons on it, presumably to prevent misuse and/or damage, which makes sense. It was also an easier, more accessible option than regular lifts because it was visible and more compact. I liked it and I felt important; I felt like my needs had been recognised (if we ignore the safety arm situation).

That is, until the day my teacher asked to borrow my remote because she wanted to use the lift to get a couple of boxes filled with heavy books up to the library. She didn't want any of the other pupils to hurt their backs … or some other excuse. The library was still a distance away from where the lift was, so they still would have had to carry the boxes for part of the way.

[RANT LOADING…]
Are you being serious right now?

We fight and advocate for literally years to get this lift into the school and functioning so that I (and those with disabilities who would follow) could gain access to an education and then you come over like, "Oh, this is convenient" and want to use it as a book courier service?! Yes, I'm just a little bitter.

These are the moments that make me so angry when I think back on my high-school experience because they made me feel like very few fucks were given about *my* wellbeing and my ability to have any sort of equitable education in that space. What makes it worse is that I was pretty much in survival mode for almost four years. My resistance was low and I gave her my remote! I'm still kind of mad at myself for not making a scene about this, but there are so many battles going on right now, so, "Whatever, dude, it doesn't matter anyway."
[RANT OVER]

My days at school consisted of fighting with boys about why they needed to carry me up the stairs every 45 minutes; hearing "you're late" every 45 minutes; not really knowing who was on my side and who was wanting to cause me strife. It's hard to tell, when there were very few people who I felt had stuck up for me in those situations. Don't get me wrong, there were a couple of people who did do this and created spaces where I felt safe. I hope these people know who they are, and know how important they were during a time of my life when I didn't feel I had a place where I belonged and felt accepted.

The overwhelming feeling I had during the first four years of high school was one of loneliness. I wasn't trying to play my disability card and manipulate the system to avoid having to do things or so that I wouldn't have to work as hard as my classmates. I was ready to do the work. I just wanted to feel seen. I didn't want to feel like my wheelchair was bigger than I was; that it was this insurmountable obstacle that the people around me couldn't get over. I wanted to feel like people understood me and saw me for my ability and not just for how I got around.

A memory that stands out for me involves an English assignment we had in Grade 9. (It was an oral and I like talking, so you'd think this would be easy for me...) We had to find song lyrics – it was okay if it was more than one song – and explain to the class why those lyrics represented ourselves or our personalities. Sounds pretty simple, right? I thought so too. But when I started looking into the songs that I was listening to and those that I felt a connection with and related to in some way, they were all kind of depressing and I didn't want people to overanalyse my song choices (like I'm doing right now) and for that to be the image people had of me; an image that I would then have had a hand in creating.

One of the songs was *Hello* by Evanescence and the lyrics of that song are pretty intense. For example:

Don't try to fix me, I'm not broken
Hello, I'm the lie living for you so you can hide.

Another song I was looking at was Kate Voegele's *Angel*, which I felt fit better with my activist side, my confident, outside-of-school self, with lines like:
I ain't got no sob story to write
But just like everyone else I'm living this life
And you don't need to win me over
And there ain't no other side to shelter me from
I belong where I decide.

I struggled for a long time with that assignment and never found songs that I thought I could speak about in relation to my life and how I felt about it. I didn't want to use songs that were overly confident and self-assured because then I'd seem pompous or arrogant (or so I thought). And yeah, maybe I'm listening to music that is a little morbid, but that doesn't mean that I'm completely depressed and don't have a life that I think is great. I still felt like I had a good grasp on who I was, and I was happy about who I was. I just didn't feel that I could be that person when I was at school. I never actually did that oral. Nobody really made an issue out of it either.

A second example was when my motorised chair had gone in for a service or something, which meant that I had to go to school in a manual chair. This shouldn't have been that big of a deal, but it felt big to me. I was in a Maths lesson and our teacher left the classroom to go and sort out some admin.

[TANGENT]
My Maths teacher was also our grade head and she was an amazing supporter. Her classroom was somewhere I felt safe because she accommodated my disability, but still recognised my ability. I realised, sitting in her class, that it wasn't actually that hard to be a supporter and that it's not that hard to call people out when they're being horrible humans.

I didn't take notes in her class because she would print them for me afterwards, so I could just listen and absorb what she was teaching. There was a group of boys who sat in the corner close to her desk and one of them said: "Why do we have to write the notes and Chaeli can just get them printed?"

She was quick to respond. I think it was intended to be an under-the-radar comment, but it didn't work out that way for him. She said, "Do your hands work perfectly? Yes? When your hands stop working as efficiently as they do now, I'll print the notes for you too."

Nobody ever commented again in her class about notes getting printed for me. In that moment, she became like a rock star to me. She took on months of anxiety from bullies and crushed it in a single sentence. When I walked past her at school I felt like I could exhale, just a little. I had a few teachers who did this for me – Maths, Biology and English in Grade 10 were the lessons I was living for.
[TANGENT OVER]

I remember that when the teacher was out of the room, a group of girls sitting behind me kept touching/pushing my wheelchair and giggling. I felt powerless. That was the day I told my parents that I wasn't going to go to school if for any reason I didn't have my motorised wheelchair.

I was called in for counselling a few times, and I had, and still have, conflicting ideas around this. At the time, I was still pretending that I was fine and perfectly happy. In some ways I appreciated it because it got me away from everyone who was giving me a hard time for 30 minutes. But it also caused a lot of panic – what if the counsellor could see right through me? I found myself stuck between wanting to feel that I could breathe without people judging me, and not wanting people to know or see that maybe I wasn't this superhuman disabled person who could overcome any and all obstacles with her positivity superpowers. Thinking about it now, that whole situation made no sense to me and actually makes me angry. I was only called in for a session 18 months after I got to high school because the counsellor was nervous about not being able to understand me. Calling me in for a session to talk about what animal I identify with (it's a llama, in case you're wondering) when I have some real issues going on in my life is not really helpful. I felt that my issues were not because of my personal life or anything that I had done. My issues were created by actions carried out by other people who didn't understand my disability, at school. Why should that have been my problem or something that I had to deal with at all? Why weren't they counselling the people who were making my school life impossible? After our slightly rocky start, that counsellor ended up becoming one of the biggest advocates for inclusion at the school, and that, to me, is a success story. I don't hold her inclusion understanding starting point against her. Would I have appreciated more understanding and support while I was at the school? For sure. The takeaway for me is that she came round and proved that people have the ability to change and expand their perspectives. It may take work and time, but it's possible.

Bullying is often understood in terms of black eyes, broken bones and bruises, but when people are constantly "attacking" you and pointing out things that you cannot change, that is a more powerful weapon than any fist. High-school bullying is often just innocent enough that it either doesn't show up on the radar or it's disregarded as harmless fun that's simply being misinterpreted. Schools need to get smarter then, I'm afraid. These years of high school made me question everything I knew about myself, and I felt invisible. (And what's worse is that the experience made me *want* to be invisible.) Many of the moments that have stayed with my psyche from high school were throwaway comments. It may seem trivial or harmless to have someone say "You're late" seven or eight times every school day, but it wore me down. I tried to just ignore it, but it's difficult to pretend it didn't happen.

My parents were told that the pupils didn't want to help me, and this may have been the main reason I was experiencing difficulties. Here's the thing: a person's attitude is shaped and guided by the ways in which a situation is framed. And schools should totally let overly hormonal 15-year-olds dictate the trajectory of the school, right? (Yes, that's sarcasm...) Surely we go to school to learn and be guided to become decent human beings? Notwithstanding puberty, of course, when everyone is supposedly developmentally appropriately awful. Keep in mind that this happens right around Grade 9, which is where we are at this point in the story. We still felt that we needed to know how much truth there was in this claim that my peers didn't want to be helpful. A survey was done shortly after this discussion took place and it wasn't really framed in a way that would make my school life easier.

It was a simple survey. It went something like this:

1. Do you want to help Chaeli? (Yes/No)
2. If yes, what are you willing to help her with?

Then there was a check list of things to tick the options that applied. (They literally tried to put my disability in a box.) It was things like carrying me up and down the stairs; transferring me between wheelchairs; getting books and stationery out of my bag; helping in Art class with supplies, etc.

3. Any other comments?

This survey was done on one of the days when I was absent. Thank goodness. That would have led to some unbearable awkwardness. I was absent from school fairly regularly. Sometimes it was because I had things to do with The Chaeli Campaign and sometimes I was at home, sick. (I think feeling sick was my body activating a self-protection mechanism.)

The survey was completed anonymously. Apparently, anonymity is protective. (Well, it didn't protect me, that's for sure.) Anonymous can also be interpreted as "I can be an ass, and nobody will know". There wasn't any meaningful follow-up discussion about it or really any action at all from the school. It was just a bomb blowing up my already-tense school experience, and everyone just seemed to carry on with their lives, like when you fill in a service satisfaction survey at a restaurant or hotel that is quickly forgotten.

The results of the survey came back, and out of the 31 pupils in my class only eight of them said they were willing to help me in any way, and nobody was willing to help with lifting or transferring me, just getting my books and stuff out of my bag and putting it back in my bag after class. That's like a 25% compassion ratio and to me that's horrendous. Then there were the additional comments that everyone could add. And we all know that teenagers really like to share their opinions. There were three main points made that we can appreciate as having some legitimacy: "We don't want to hurt Chaeli", "We don't want to hurt ourselves" and "It's not fair if we're the only ones doing it." This makes sense to me at some level, but I also feel these are thoughts that didn't really consider my feelings. I was in a position where I needed to be reflective and have empathy for my classmates, when they weren't expected to do the same. My views and feelings weren't given the same consideration.

The school was upset, not because the sentiment towards me exposed by the survey was deplorable, but because the results of that survey were shared with me. They felt that it was irresponsible of my parents to have shared the results with me because they were so negative and might affect my self-esteem... Thanks for your input. Interesting that my wellbeing and happiness suddenly became important, when this concern was completely lacking throughout that whole process. I was winded, and my world was sufficiently rocked. A one-page survey confirmed my fears and feelings that when I was at school, I was virtually unsupported. I appreciate that I was told and exposed to the reality of my situation and the magnitude of the battle I had ahead of me. Instead of going back to school like some idiot ostrich that's had its head in the sand, oblivious to anything that has happened around it, I could use that information to become a detective to somehow figure out my new school strategy. That worked for about a year.

My strategy involved a lot of absenteeism and avoidance. Breaktime was the worst. I didn't really have many friends at school. I didn't get invited to any parties or get-togethers. I wasn't in any of the cliques that had established themselves within the first week of high school that are basically impenetrable after this. I also developed strategies to be as self-sufficient as I could be, knowing that my peers were not interested in helping me. I started using a lever arch file where I kept my work for all my subjects instead of having separate books for each subject, so I didn't have to ask for help with that in every class. I also stopped putting any meaningful effort into my schoolwork.

My activities, like wheelchair dancing and my activism, didn't really fit into the school's recognition system, so my life was outside of school. I often wonder why my absenteeism wasn't brought up by the school in a more serious way, but at the same time I was in survival mode, so I was also okay with nobody saying anything. If they brought it up, I'd have to confront my issues and I wasn't ready for that, so I was on board with being unnoticed just then. I had made myself believe I was okay with being invisible. I had convinced myself and rationalised that it was a temporary thing – I only needed to be invisible for six hours a day.

[TANGENT]
I think one of the greatest moments, if not *the* greatest moment, of my high-school career happened in our homeroom lesson at the start of a school day. It was after the survey debacle and we had worked out a new plan for how I would get to my upstairs classes. Enter Jason.

Jason was Tarryn's boyfriend at the time (he is now her husband) and we asked him if he would be keen to help me get upstairs, and in the process hopefully change the perception and reframe what it was like to help me. The plan was that Jason would have my timetable and come in when I needed help getting up or down the stairs and then he would leave again. Jason was coaching cricket at the time, so his schedule was mostly flexible.

So on this day I knew he was coming, but nobody else did. I was nervous about how people around me would respond. He arrived to introduce himself to my homeroom teacher, walked into our class holding his bike helmet in his hand (this caught the boys' attention) and, before introducing himself, he came over to me and kissed me on the cheek (which caught the girls' attention). He interrupted the entire flow of the lesson and it was everything. He shook my teacher's hand and said, "Hi, I'm Jason. I'll be assisting Chaeli with the stairs for the rest of the term." Then he looked at me and said, "I'll be back later when you need me."

Jaws hit the floor and it was glorious.
[TANGENT OVER]

I'm grateful that I haven't ever really had that "Why me?" response to things linked to my disability, and my school experience was no different. I never thought my life would be better if I wasn't disabled. I just couldn't understand why they felt the need to be so nasty and point out my disability so blatantly when my needs were pretty obvious in my mind. *Plays Taylor Swift's Mean at full volume.*
There were things that happened that could have been seen as indicators that all was not well; that could have changed the trajectory of my school life. When I applied to run for Representative Council of Learners (RCL), I wasn't allowed to because I had missed too many school days. This apparently meant that I wasn't reliable enough for the responsibilities of RCL. Granted, I had missed a lot of school – 40 days or something. This could have been a profound moment of intervention and support. It was an opportunity to engage with me and find out what was going on and to get me out of the dark place in which I found myself, but it ended up being another school experience where I felt excluded and my skills unappreciated.

I had regular meltdowns throughout high school. Most of the time I wasn't able to communicate my thoughts because crying and hyperventilating are not conducive to communicating big feelings. So, Mom would ask me to write down my thoughts and feelings, and email them to her (gotta love technology). We could then talk about it later, when I'd gathered myself. This worked for me because it gave me time to process everything in my brain and have an outlet, so I didn't keep *everything* bottled up inside me. I started writing these emails when I was about 14 years old, and Mom has kept them. She's always been the queen archivist, for times like this. Some of them are pretty intense. She didn't keep them for this particular purpose, but because this is about honesty and being vulnerable and real, why not share those thoughts here?

(July 2009 – Grade 9)

I'm not important to any of those people. I'm not a priority on anybody's list. I don't want to be the centre of attention, but I want people to care. I want to be in a place where I matter.

You said that I mustn't blame the kids because the teachers didn't do all that they could. The teachers weren't the ones who said those things about me. Those people are not my friends. I can't be friends with people who don't understand me or accept me and think I'm a cripple.

You expect me to pay no mind to what they say, but I can't. I don't have that kind of emotional strength.

I remember always stressing about having to walk from home to school, but never worrying about the journey home. I always wanted my parents to drive me there, even though we live only about 800m from the school. I think it's because school created anxiety for me – not the work, but the people who surrounded me – and if we drove there, I had less time to talk or think myself into a space of not wanting to go at all. Eventually, that stopped working and the dam wall of my emotions broke on the first day of term three in my Grade 11 year. When we'd reached week three of me refusing to go to school, I was taken seriously and my extended meltdown became a statement. Don't think that my parents didn't try to help. Trust me, they tried so hard. One day, Mom managed to get me dressed in my uniform, into the car and into the parking lot. I even made it to the back door of the school before I turned into an anxious puddle of tears and was swiftly taken back home. But that was the moment I also started taking myself seriously and believing that my feelings and emotions were real and valid. I stopped denying that I had them. It was difficult to admit to other people, but even more so to myself, that I wasn't happy where I was. I deserved better.

People didn't understand how I was feeling. I wanted to explain but I also didn't want it to seem like I was setting up for a pity party. I wanted my experiences to be helpful to other people. Maybe a lot of people were feeling alone and were scared to expose their vulnerabilities. I was scared, too, but I couldn't keep it inside any more, and even though it would open me up to critique, I had to share how I was feeling, so I wrote a letter. I had been meaning to start writing it for a while, when I was having my meltdown, and hadn't found the strength to admit to myself the depth of the situation I was in or find the words to express those emotions eloquently. I was compelled to write after an experience that solidified for me the urgency of my feelings and the need to share them. One Saturday we went to a conference focused on inclusive education with the title "Making Ordinary Schools Special"; I think it was run by the Department of Education. We were presenting on our work through The Chaeli Campaign and our personal experiences.

When we arrived, we found out that our presentation was upstairs, which was in and of itself not a problem, but the lift was out of order, so I had to be carried up three flights of stairs. Usually this wouldn't have been a major issue, but considering my fragile emotional state, it was one more thing where I had to make a plan; one more time that my needs weren't considered. In a space where everyone is preaching about being aware, considerate and accommodating of anyone's different challenges and needs, that was especially hard for me to absorb. It was also hard because it was a conference about how inclusive education is possible and where people were all talking about their solutions and successes. There I was, having a shitty experience of education as a disabled person, having refused to go to school for almost a month, in the middle of a breakdown. I didn't feel like I was the poster child for inclusive education. I think our presentation truly reflected how hard it can be, and showed that inclusion isn't the easy option. And honestly, at that point I was an advocate for being a hermit and never leaving home again, so it wasn't necessarily a great time for my activist self.

When we got home after the conference, I had the urge to start writing and I disappeared into my bedroom for about four hours and finished my open letter. It took this long because my first few versions were probably the bitchiest things I've ever written. These versions were important for me to just vent my feelings. When I was finished writing, I figured out who I was going to send it to – the headmaster and deputy, the student heads and the governing body of the school. I emailed it. I remember feeling so empowered when I clicked on "Send" and I rolled out of my room feeling like such a boss. My parents and sister were sitting outside on the stoep and I sat at the door and said, "I sent it" and they all nodded and told me I had done a good job and that they were proud of me for using my voice in this way. Fifteen minutes later we were getting ready to eat supper and the magnitude of what I had just done hit me hard. I instantly felt sick and went pale. I remember sitting in the kitchen, leaning on Dad, bursting into tears and crying so hard I was shaking, terrified about what would happen when I got to school on Monday.

After a panic-stricken weekend and a fair amount of crying I didn't go to school on Monday. Instead, I spent the day eating a whole lot of everything and conjuring up every possible response I could have to anyone who had read my letter. I had them stockpiled like I was preparing for the end of the world. I think I was, in my own way, and I thought that that letter would change my life as I knew it. It did, just not in the way I had expected. When I arrived at school the following day, with my false confidence, I expected a barrage of responses. I was ready for their disgust, defensive comments and anger, maybe a supportive gesture or gaze somewhere, but there was nothing. Nobody said or did anything. It was just your regular Tuesday. Was it arrogant of me to think that anyone cared what I had to say? That was harder than any of the situations I'd prepared myself for, because it confirmed in that moment that all the things I was feeling – the things I had convinced myself weren't real, just the consequence of my overthinking and overanalysis – were in fact true. It confirmed that how I was feeling, my words and my value remained unseen and seemingly unimportant to anyone that I was spending most of my waking hours with. It didn't matter. I rode around school that day totally lost and confused. What else could I do? After going around unnoticed for a few more days, and being overtly ignored, I knew that I couldn't stay in that space a minute longer. I called my parents, and someone came to fetch me to take me home.

There's always time for a good metaphor to give perspective, right? You'd think so, but it's not always appreciated. Sometimes it's hit and miss. For example...

Mom, trying to convince me on day 12 or something of my school strike that going to school would be in my best interest, said, "Chaeli, you can't fight the dragons unless you face the dragons." That is a good metaphor and may even classify as superhero sidekick pep talk level motivational. Except, not on this day. Not for me. You know what I had to say about it?

Fuck the dragons.

There are too many dragons. I don't have the energy or resistance any more to deal with all of them. Maybe I could fight one, but not when there are 30-plus dragons in a closed space, and every 30 to 45 minutes the dragons change shape and position. It's too much. I'd also never seen a woman taking on a giant-ass dragon by herself (down with the patriarchy for making me question whether I can take on a dragon – pshh!), so I wasn't on board with this metaphor, as I'm sure you're aware by now.

[FLASHBACK]
Years after I had finished high school my mom and I were driving past my old school on the way home one day and I looked at the school building, reminiscing. I told Mom, "I think I checked out of here a long time before I left." She found this to be quite a profound statement, and it led to quite a deep, hectic conversation in the car when we got home. We tend to have these intense conversations and spend hours talking in the car, parked in our driveway.
[FLASHBACK OVER]

I am constantly grateful for my disability. Yes, there are definitely times when I'm frustrated by the situations it gets me into and my body lets me down regularly. I'm grateful for my disability because it also saves me from a lot of things. My disability makes me consider things differently. I don't have control over a lot of things in my life, so I choose not to do certain things where I would have less control and be more vulnerable. My physical ability (or limitations in this case) would not allow me to be reckless in typical ways or engage in certain destructive behaviours. I would need assistance and accomplices. People would then know and find out.

While we were sitting in our parked car in our driveway, Mom told me that if I had been able-bodied and having the experiences or feelings I was having during my early high-school career, she would have been worried about me hurting myself or doing something worse. I didn't say anything because I think there was more truth to that statement than I was ready to admit to anyone. Even to myself. I don't think her worry would have been misplaced; it wasn't too far from how I was feeling and where my headspace was.

The realisation hit me like a pair of shoes falling out of the sky and hitting me in the face – unexpected and confusing. I realised right then that during my first years in high school I was in a very dark place emotionally, not able to see a way out of that darkness. I know that it was a dark time because I remember feeling so frustrated that I couldn't do anything; I couldn't rebel and find ways of escaping from where I was. I felt stuck. I wasn't even able to do something drastic. (Because, you know, you have to be drastic to be taken seriously.) I didn't know how to make them see and understand how I was feeling. I wanted to be able to do something drastic and force myself out of my invisibility and force those who had hurt me to see how they had affected me, but I couldn't. My disability wouldn't let me. My disability very possibly saved my life.

So I'll say it again. I'm grateful for my disability and the incredible life it has brought me.

I'm not sharing these stories as a form of revenge and I'm not holding out for apologies. I'm sharing these stories for myself, as a self-care tool, to get to a point where I can let go of high school. I know this because even now, almost a decade after leaving, whenever I go there, I know that everyone (apart from some of the teachers) who was there when I was has moved on, but those memories live in the walls. I still feel the most intense anxiety. I can't go through those passages without turning back into that insecure teenager I was in that space. I'm not there yet, but I'll get there.

Many things are said by those who are meant to help children who are struggling in school (teachers, counsellors, headmasters); people who are meant to recognise when children need help. Most of the time it's not deliberate, people just don't realise what's happening. "She seems fine; very positive", "That's not bullying" and "She copes so well with everything" are some of the comments I regularly heard. Alongside the rationalised mission to become invisible, I got really good at looking busy. If I could pull off not having to engage with anyone for a few hours, it felt like a win to me. With my schoolwork, I was doing virtually nothing in class. When you're working on a laptop, nobody questions what you're doing. I mastered justifying why other people didn't understand my disability and giving them excuses before they could find them for themselves. Maybe I was just a good actor. Maybe I was waiting for someone to notice that I was full of shit and call my bluff. I don't know.

If you were in my year, or were around when I was, and remember me at this point of high school, I hope you can have a better understanding of where I was at and what I was feeling and experiencing. If you can see yourselves in some of these stories, I hope that you recognise that your words have power and leave lasting imprints. If you were one of the people who created a safe space for me, thank you. You were bubbles of oxygen when I felt like I was drowning.

Those years in high school made me feel really vulnerable. I don't like thinking about the stories that take me back to that place because I'm not that person any more. I'm not as scared of people pointing out my disability as I used to be; I own it more now. This is probably because my fuck-you mechanism was well honed over this period and I have more supportive people around me in my day-to-day life, so the issues that existed and were seen as the biggest deal then just aren't any more. That being said, the fact that I survived high school and made it out semi-okay doesn't make my experiences acceptable. I still get completely anxious if I have to go back there for any reason, even if I'm just sitting in the parking lot. I'm still triggered when people say something seemingly mundane and harmless, because all of the experiences I've had live on in my mind. And I have moved on and forwards, but at the same time I think they have had a bigger impact than we initially appreciated.

I'd like to be able to say that my disability had a minimal impact on my education, but that would be a blatant lie. I'd like to say that my educators and peers didn't see me differently and that this wasn't a factor in how I was treated, but they did and it was. I've accepted that in my life and I want to use my experiences, although they were negative, to show the reality of how truly trying an inclusive education can be. It's not the easy option, that's for sure. I wouldn't have it any other way, though. The crappy, difficult moments have bigger, stronger claws that take hold, and any positive memories have to fight harder to be seen. You can take whatever metaphor you like from that.

Many people have experienced a life-altering moment. These moments of clarity can be profound and big, like you're under a spotlight; and sometimes they're tiny interactions nobody else notices that make every thought you have been trying to keep quiet come flooding in and you can no longer avoid them.

It wasn't a single event that created this experience for me, but there was definitely a moment of clarity when I knew I needed to get out of the situation.

I knew that people had read my letter, not because anything crazy happened but because I felt that their eyes were different when they looked at me. Maybe I was projecting. Maybe nothing had changed. I begrudgingly went to school that day. I was trying to do the invisible wheelchair-user thing when I'd just sent an open letter to the entire leadership of the school. It was the middle of the school day and I was deep in survival mode. I got out of the lift and made my way to one of my only independently accessible lessons of the day. I was running late. Obviously. The headmaster was in the passage and I said, "Good morning, Sir" as he walked towards me. I was expecting the usual reciprocal response, but I didn't get it. Instead, he heard and saw me, looked me in the eye, said nothing, looked away, then walked around me. I was stunned and incensed and hurt that he wouldn't look 16-year-old me in the eye because I had written a letter talking about my feelings.

This was my life-altering moment. It took me almost four years to reach this point of no return. It sounds ironic, as I've been an activist for pretty much my whole life, but that was the moment I started speaking for myself (and with myself), thinking of my own wellbeing as opposed to thinking of all the possible challenges that lay ahead if I had to move schools. I decided that I just couldn't be there any more and was willing to look at all other options. We found the best solution, after my initial coping mechanism of crying and Nutella. Moving schools was the only option that was acceptable to me and it made all the difference.

It's crazy to think that the most amazing and worst things in my life were happening at the same time. While I was living through the hardest time at school, preparations were happening for us to travel to the Netherlands, because I had been chosen as the 2011 recipient of the International Children's Peace Prize. This was where my double-life experience felt all the more serious and real.

Once again, we made a big decision and in the short space of two weeks I had changed schools. At this stage I was a peer mentor (a Grade 11 student who mentors Grade 8 students about dealing with high school). I recognise that given the above stories, I possibly didn't have the best mindset to be advising anyone about anything. Anyway, when I told the teacher in charge of that Grade 8 class that I was leaving at the end of the week, she was shocked and told me that I should have mentioned earlier that I was leaving, as they would have thrown a going-away party. While I can (now) appreciate the sentiment, at the time I felt it was a case of a little bit too little, too late. I know that going through what I did made it easier for those who came after me, but sometimes it's hard to feel like a casualty in the cause for the greater good. I know that when you're one of the first or only people doing something new or something deemed outside the norm, you're automatically a pioneer and a trailblazer. It's hard to be that – there's so much pressure in it and sometimes you don't want to be. Mostly you just want to be accepted and feel that you belong somewhere.

Arrangements had been made and I was given a full scholarship to a private school. I then found myself in a new, very different place. It was a place where my disability wasn't the barrier it had been before. It was just the thing that made my support needs unique. Don't get me wrong, I would have preferred not to have had such a negative experience in my first three-

and-a-half years of high school, but we learnt many lessons in that negativity. We could then say, "We tried this and it didn't work so well" – and that led to finding better solutions. I wasn't treated like a burden, or as though I were taking up somebody else's space. The expectations were explicit. "Chaeli is one of us, and we support one another"; "You are not going to wait for Chaeli to ask for help – you will be aware and offer to help". It took me a long time to trust in these intentions. I was so used to people not wanting to help me and fighting with people about carrying me up the stairs, that when my peers were offering assistance without being asked, I didn't believe they were being genuine. I still carry these thoughts with me, but I'm learning to let them go.

I remember my first day. It was a Friday...

Wait, let's go back a bit. I had stopped going to my previous school at this point, so my schedule was wide open to figure out how I was going to navigate my new school environment. It was a whirlwind week. On the Tuesday, I was asked to come to the school to chat to the staff. All the staff. I was intimidated and I wasn't sure what to say. When I asked, I was told, "Just tell them what you expect of them." Um, what?! I wasn't used to being able to share my expectations of my educators and leading the conversation on the support I needed. Then, on the Wednesday, I was invited to chat to my new peers, all the Grade 11 students, about some things to be aware of and ways that they could help or support me. There were a few people that I had gone to primary school with, so I had some friendly, familiar faces in the crowd. When I asked whether anyone had any questions, I realised that I was in a more positive place. One of the boys asked me what the plan was for when it rains because the school is very open, with not a lot of coverage. I said that I guessed we would figure it out when it started raining. He told me that he would hold an umbrella for me if necessary.

It's in the small things. In that moment, I felt seen.

Back to my first day. It was the Friday of this whirlwind week and, as luck would have it, it was raining. It was August – I remember because I had my birthday two or three weeks later – and August is pretty much always raining. This was not regular rain, though, it was drenching-downpour, burst-cloud, grab-your-paddle rain. So that was super helpful. When I arrived at school in this weather I was nervous but mostly excited because

I knew it was the start of something. I was nervous because I didn't want to electrocute myself by going through a puddle with my wheelchair. (I'm not even sure this is possible – the chair would probably just stop working. I'll investigate this...) That would have made a less than ideal first impression. This was apart from all the regular stress of a first day of school. I had been told to go to reception, where I would get my timetable and everything I needed, so that was my plan. However, while I was being carried to my wheelchair, which was parked behind the car under the boot to prevent it from getting unnecessarily drenched (our car's boot acts as a handy shelter in times like this), two boys from my grade ran across the parking lot with umbrellas to help me to my first class.

Mom sat in the car sobbing for a good 10 minutes after this. (She says it wasn't that long, but I'm not so sure.) After witnessing me feeling so lost, so unsupported and so desperate to be accepted, seeing two young boys who were essentially strangers be so accommodating and caring was just too much for her. I think this is where we all realised we could exhale. Thinking about this moment in my life, I realise that my experiences have an impact on the people around me in very significant ways. In a different way from how they impact me, but significant nonetheless.

Something that sticks in my memory was being asked to give a presentation in assembly on my trip to the Netherlands to accept the International Children's Peace Prize. I was used to giving talks because of our work with The Chaeli Campaign, but this was different. I had worked hard throughout my high-school career to blend in, to be as unnoticeable and invisible as possible. Now I was being asked to promote myself and claim recognition. I was *stressing*! I was wearing my blazer and it felt like it was a million degrees Celsius. A group of boys lifted me onto the stage and I was terrified. I wasn't terrified of speaking and sharing stories. I knew I could do that. I was afraid of the potential judgement from my peers. I thought they would see it as me bragging and trying to sound like a big deal. That was a fear based on my previous experiences. But when I finished my presentation, I said "thank you" and all of a sudden applause became a standing ovation that was led by my fellow matrics. I wasn't ready for that. If there's one thing that really triggers me, it's solidarity. I wasn't prepared for that level of appreciation and support. I don't think my peers realised what a big moment that was for me. So, I just want to say thank you for helping me feel that I belonged and that the experiences I had before were not reflective of my worth. Thank you for creating a space where I could find my voice again. A place where I learnt how to use my voice again. A place where I could be my full self.

Writing this part of my story has been hard. It's been tough going back into the memories that I clearly tried to bury somewhere deep inside myself. Maybe I'm not as over high school as I thought I was. I'll probably never fully let go of these experiences, and I think that's okay. Going through that craziness has moulded me into who I am now, with all my flaws and complexes. I can go through awful things and I can still believe that people will rise to the occasion of being the person you need them to be, to support you when you need them and to let you shine when you need to. Sometimes it takes a second (or a decade) to find the people who you are meant to share your life stories with; the people who understand you and accept you with all your complicated feelings, and you can just be who you are without stressing about anything; the people who offer to carry some of your baggage for you when it gets heavy. In my experience, they've been worth the wait.

TIME FOR BIG SCHOOL – NOW I HAVE TO BE A GROWN-UP?

As I mentioned earlier, education is a big deal for my parents, so it was a non-negotiable that Erin and I studied further. Erin got her degree from Vega and I had always seen myself studying at the University of Cape Town (UCT). When I finished high school, I did just that. I didn't consider other options because I had set my mind and heart on UCT. I did have a mild meltdown when there was a technical glitch with my application and I had no Plan B. Thankfully it was all sorted out and I was going to be an Ikey!

I was so excited to go to university, but it can also be a super stressful time. I like having a plan, so I read the prospectus obsessively, highlighting courses that sounded cool and changing my mind a million times. This uncertainty continued throughout my undergrad degree. I changed my majors five times. By the time I had earned my Bachelor of Social Science majoring in Politics and Social Development in 2015, I had done courses in Politics, Social Development, Anthropology, Sociology, Public Policy, Gender Studies, Linguistics and Philosophy. I almost had a triple major with Anthropology (I loved it so much), but when I failed the Medical Anthropology course in my second year, I would have had to extend my degree by a year to get the credits. So I decided that I didn't need to be an overachiever right then. I'm well-rounded, people.

I realised early – in the first week – that university is very different from high school. I can break down this realisation into three big ideas.

The first is that there's so much freedom, in so many ways. Freedom to be who you are (and figure out who that is), to make decisions and to choose who you spend your time with. Building friendship circles was easier for me because there was more freedom to find people who align with me in terms of values and purpose. I grew deeper friendships that I feel safe and secure in, in a way I didn't feel when I was in high school. Living in res, away from home, was another level of freedom I'd never experienced before.

[TANGENT]
I was the first person to stay in the residence who had a disability severe enough to necessitate a personal-care assistant. The day I moved in was insane – months earlier we had scheduled a knee surgery and it happened to be the day before move-in day. I had the surgery on the Monday, was

discharged from hospital on the Tuesday, went home, packed some outfits and a few other essentials into a suitcase and proceeded to move into res with my new personal-care assistant, Nthabiseng. I was not fazed. I have had many surgeries, and we knew how to handle everything.

[TANGENT OVER]

Second is taking responsibility for everything in my life. This was especially true in terms of work things. All of a sudden, I had to manage my own schedule, and nobody was checking up on me, making sure I was getting everything done. It was all up to me. That was a major lesson for me, especially staying away from home. The realisation of autonomy was real and it was pretty immediate.

The third and biggest thing that was different at university was how my disability was treated and understood. My experiences at high school had taught me that my disability was a major factor for people defining me in their minds based mostly on what they could see of my disability; that they didn't need to look any further. As a way to combat this attitude I'd learnt to act pre-emptively. I had an elevator pitch, where I spoke about my disability (diagnosis and stuff) first to get it out there. I would always emphasise that my disability wasn't the biggest deal (even though it definitely *is* a key determining factor), so in a way that sort of brushed over it, as if it weren't a key role player in my life. I thought people would appreciate that more than if I were to fully embrace my disability in all its glory.

I was completely unprepared when I arrived at university for orientation week and my carefully crafted elevator pitch was unnecessary because nobody asked me about my disability at all. We were working off different assumptions – I was assuming that my disability would matter to people because for years it had always been the main thing anyone asked about, but the new people I was meeting at university were working off the assumption that because I was at university, I had earned my place to be there based on merit, and my disability wasn't a factor in that happening. People didn't care about what my disability was; that was a conversation we could have later. I had spent so much time thinking about how people might respond to the fact that I was disabled that when I was asked questions like "What are you majoring in?" I didn't have *any* solid answers. It is perfectly okay for people to ask other non-disability-related questions and be interested in learning about the magnitude of other things that make me, me. People can see and appreciate my disability and still care more about the rest of my story.

It was good for me to learn this early on in my university career. Obviously, university has its own struggles and stresses (especially when I'm in a wheelchair and my university campus is located on a mountain). It took a second for me to learn all the alternative routes around campus. It's always the long way round for the accessible route. (This is the case everywhere, not just at my university.) My friends were always confused when they walked with me to class because often we would go in and out of different buildings and take lifts to different levels to get to where we wanted to be. If you need to get somewhere fast, don't ask me for directions. I'll send you on an accessible adventure.

PANIC ATTACK...
(I decided to write through a panic attack, and this is what came out...)

I live with anxiety. It lives with me. I exist in a body that constantly disagrees with my mind, and when I try to exert some authority or power, my body throws it right back. In these moments, when I smile and make a joke, I laugh first, while my pencil case falls to the floor and my highlighters roll down the lecture theatre steps, making sure that I'm not making anyone too uncomfortable. In these moments (and all the others) is where my anxiety lives. I'm not always sure it's around ... maybe it's sleeping. Let's try not to wake it up.

I exist in a world that isn't designed for me and every day I'm honing my skills as an architect. Often I'm confronted with doors. They're not slammed in my face, they're just closed. Anxiety hides here. In the crevices and corners and the bookshelves of my mind where I'm keeping all those (all-but) forgotten throwaway comments that they thought I couldn't hear. I pretend not to hear them, or try to use sassy comebacks as doorstops. Oh, but she's funny! The laughter is there to mask my heart rate. Anxiety is the wind that blows the window closed, taking all the oxygen from the room I'm occupying.

I live in that weird space between invisibility and being too loud where, when I roll into a room, everybody notices me because I take up a bit more space than they were prepared for, but at the same time people don't always remember I'm there.

"Oh, sorry, I didn't see you there." I'm right here. Is it because I'm below your eyeline or is your perspective of the world just tinted with filters like green screens so you can add context later? I'm positive that these things can and will change in time, but sometimes I'm tired – trying to unblur lines and unpack all of these complicated situations and issues that I'm not always sure I even understand. Sometimes I'm angry and then being angry makes me sad, and then I feel guilty that I'm angry and sad, and how can I be these things when my life could really be so much harder? These are the moments when I doubt everything. Even the feelings I'm feeling. Are these actually my feelings or am I projecting feelings from the world about me? Is this even projecting?

TAKE A BREATH...
(Use the three-minute rule when necessary.)

KEEP BREATHING.

...I have spent many years at university unlearning the negative ideas around my disability that I learnt in high school. This is an ongoing process.

I think there are few things worse than that first tutorial of the semester where you "get to know one another better", and living through those awkward "give a character trait with the first letter of your name" activities. Then suddenly I've forgotten every word that begins with a C. Orientation week is much like this. I understand that it's important to create opportunities to connect with new people in our new environment, but every time I have to take part in an ice-breaker, I die a little inside.

When I applied for university, it was suggested that I should register for an extended degree and have a lighter course load, so that I wasn't overwhelmed or "too stressed". This annoyed me immensely. I was coming from a context of spending most of my school career in a mainstream environment, coping just fine working at the same pace as my non-disabled peers. Why should university be any different? So I registered for the typical number of courses to graduate after the standard three years for an undergraduate degree. I argued that if I ever felt overwhelmed, I could drop courses and then register for an extended degree. It was important for me to give it a go. I didn't know anybody who was relaxed and stress-free during university, and I didn't see why I should have a different experience. Except the first three weeks of first year, when I hadn't yet realised that I was supposed to self-regulate my work and my deadlines. This was swiftly followed by a wave of panic and immense stress, when I suddenly realised that I had about five assignments due and I'd done barely any reading or work of any recognisable value. Wake-up call of note.

GOOD LUCK FOR THE EXAMS?

One of my approaches to life is "what's meant to be will be" and I've always applied this to exam strategies too. I recognise it's probably not the best strategy when it comes to exams. But when applying this strategy, you have to know that crying is an ever-present possibility.

The release of exam timetables has always been a source of anxiety for me because I am notoriously unlucky when it comes to exam timetables. My exams were always placed hideously close together and, given my above-mentioned exam strategy, this is obviously highly problematic.

Take my final matric exam timetable, for example. My first couple of weeks were so chilled, with one or two exams each week, and they were the easier ones. But then, the last week of the exam series had basically all of my learning papers and I wrote six exams in five days. These are released pretty early, so you can have your meltdown and gather your emotions ahead of time. Good plan.

It became a bit of a joke because each time I finished an exam in that week from hell, as my teachers helped me pack my bag, instead of saying goodbye they would say, "See you tomorrow." It was insane, but we made it. My last day of matric exams (both Business Studies papers) began with crisis and ended with 2pm shots at the sports club. That morning, someone had organised a memorial run, and the route blocked the school's entrance, making me late. I was revising and crying in the car as we sat in the not-at-all-moving traffic. I think my whole Business Studies class was in the traffic too.

After this hideousness I thought my bad luck with exams was over. It wasn't. Fast-forward to my first exam series of university. University exams are so different from school exams. In my courses, the work wasn't divided into different papers. The papers simply covered everything you had learnt over the whole semester. I checked my exam timetable and I was scheduled to write three exams in a week. It ended up being relatively okay, though. [TANGENT]

I wrote my first and last Philosophy exam in that session. I still don't know how I passed that course and I'm still convinced that there was an administrative error, but I'll take it. Maybe I understood more than I thought I did... From the first week of Introduction to Philosophy I was completely confused, and I knew that philosophy as a degree option was just not on the cards for me. I wanted to drop it, but I had missed the window to drop courses without incurring a cost for changing courses, and my parentals weren't about to pay for my indecisiveness. So, I was doing Introduction to Philosophy. I think I took too long to realise I didn't like it because I always want to give something the benefit of the doubt – I figured that I just wasn't used to university standards and it would become more understandable to me as I settled in. I was convinced that it would get better. Sadly, in my case none of the above turned out to be true. I like clarity and answers, and I like it when people say what they think. You don't get this from philosophy. I can deal with looking at a situation from various perspectives and a lot of my other courses did this, but I felt that philosophy looked at all perspectives, all of the time, and you don't get clear answers to any of your questions. For me, it's important to state your position and then you can go from there towards whatever you're trying to get to – whether it's common ground or whatever else.

I remember being completely overtired in one of the lectures and suddenly philosophy made sense to me. I realised in that moment that if I had to be this tired in order to excel at this course, I wasn't going to make it through my three-year degree. So, we weren't a great match and at the end of the semester we parted ways.
[TANGENT OVER]

Nothing too dramatic happened during those exams. It was an intense time, but I wasn't overwhelmed. I was feeling pretty good about my academic prowess and was ready to take on the second semester of first year. I changed my courses based on a strong dislike for some of them. I was content with my choices, until I looked up my exam schedule for the end of the year. It was literally impossible to have a worse timetable. I took four courses. I wrote the exams for all of them in two days. That's four university exams in 48 hours. That's just ridiculous.

I couldn't quite believe that it could be accurate, so I checked it a million times. I was in denial. Every time I clicked on "refresh" I was hoping for an updated timetable, but it never happened. I felt it was unrealistic to expect to do well in these exams because where was there any time for me to breathe, let alone learn and absorb knowledge? When I queried it and asked if there could be an adjustment or accommodation (remember the people who told me to do an extended degree to avoid stress? Those same people) I was told that they couldn't really help me because technically there was no clash. If there had been a time overlap, they would have been able to adjust my timetable. Somehow, I passed all the exams.

My insane timetable meant I was finished with all my exams in the first week and was then on holiday. It all worked out in the end because I had been nominated for the World of Children Youth Award and the ceremony was taking place in New York the following week, so I was able to go to New York to receive the award in person. It was intense and timing was tight (very on brand for us) and in order to be in time for the ceremony we had to book our flights for as soon as possible after my exams. I wrote my Politics exam at 5pm that Tuesday and finished at 7pm. Mom and Dad picked me up from my exam, bags already packed, and we headed straight to the airport. I was exhausted, but figured it was fine because I had 16 hours to sleep on the plane. My body was finished and had no more energy to resist anything. I got bronchitis on our way to New York and lost my voice. I was just able to give my acceptance speech (with a disclaimer that my illness had nothing to do with my disability). We met some of the most amazing people on that trip. We also learnt the valuable lesson that we cannot spend less than a week in a place when it takes three days to get to that place.

I don't know about anyone else, but I have never felt I was on top of anything when it came to my coursework. This trend followed me from my schooldays. At university, though, we'd be three days into the semester and I would already feel as though I was five weeks behind. I was constantly sleep-deprived and having internal debates about the value of time to work on assignments versus grade percentages. I tended to find for the former, taking the 10% deduction for late submission to make sure whatever I submitted was just a little better. Honestly, this is probably me justifying my deeply rooted procrastination practices. Generally, my referencing would take me an age (because it's the worst thing about university) and I'd start an essay a day or two before it was due.

I failed twice at university (shit happens) and both courses were important/required for the awarding of the degree in those majors. One was Medical Anthropology and the other was Comparative Politics. It wouldn't have been too bad, but I took those courses in the same semester, so it meant I effectively passed 50% of my courses. I don't know what happened. If I'm being honest I could have worked harder on those, but alas, it is what it is. What hurt my soul was that Comparative Politics was a mandatory course, so I had to take it again, and after I had retaken and passed it, the Politics Department changed the requirements and took it off the mandatory course list. I'm sure you can imagine what went through my mind and the expression on my face. So stoked.

I did all the things students do. I stayed out late, arriving back at res just in time to get ready for my 8am lecture (sometimes hung-over). I did my work, but also found shortcuts. (Sometimes the shortcut is also not doing the work.) I missed lectures (I may have skipped them) and had friends send notes when I didn't go. If you ask anyone about their university days, I'm prepared to bet the first three things that come to mind have nothing to do with classes or anything academic. Why should my university experience be any different because I'm disabled?

I completed my undergrad and continued to do my honours in Social Policy and Management, which worked really well with everything I was doing and learning with The Chaeli Campaign. I must say, postgraduate studies are a different beast! It's a very different kind of struggle you're signing up for. When you reach postgrad, people have higher expectations (of course, this makes sense) because you're supposed to know stuff and be able to do stuff by now. Obviously I know stuff, otherwise I wouldn't have been accepted to do the degree, but imposter syndrome is a real thing. It kicks in hard when you reach that level of academia.

The journey continues and I'm happy I've had these experiences, and am proud of how far I've come in gaining an education that in a way many doubted was possible (me too, sometimes). It wasn't always easy, and many years were a huge struggle, but it has led to a place where I feel confident and empowered by my achievements. I've learnt not to listen to the haters or allow them to dictate how I respond to negative situations. All of that has brought incredible people into my story, and that's where I'm choosing to focus my energy.

Chapter 4
Scar tissue

Our bodies are important, powerful, phenomenal creations. They are, after all, the vessel we use to get through life and navigate the world. They carry everything we experience – physically, emotionally, all of it – and I've learnt that there is a balance (not that I've mastered said balance) between pushing your body to its physical limits and giving it space to breathe and lighten the load of the weight it carries for us. That's a massive job. Life is a crazy, intense experience that we all share in some way or another, and it leaves its marks in some recognisable ways, like scar tissue.

Scar tissue... I've thought about this phenomenon a lot, in many different contexts, and I went on a journey of discovery to find some deeper meaning. Admittedly, it was a procrastination strategy, but it led to a pretty decent conversation with myself. I did what most people do when they start looking for information – I headed straight to Google. I searched for "scar tissue" and found this on *spokanepainfree.com*. It's pretty much just a medical understanding...

Internal scar tissue affects every part of your body including your organs, muscles and connective tissue. Scar tissue forms when the body undergoes trauma or inflammation of your cells and tissue. In some cases, scar tissues link together to form an adhesion, which is a band of scar tissue. The adhesion connects two internal parts, which may restrict movement or hinder things like organs from performing their intended functions. Often people with adhesions experience no symptoms or complications.

I don't believe that scars are just the body's physical response to a trauma or happening. It's bigger than that. We all go through things that are emotionally difficult and we have emotional scars that are equally as heavy and hard to heal as the physical stuff (sometimes more so). They are always there, just under the surface, building layers of protection, which can be a good or bad thing, depending on what they attach to and how serious the "injuries" are. Sometimes we need other people to help us to heal or find ways around the things that have hurt us, and that's okay. Things take time to heal and rebuild, but that's the beauty of the body. It can rejuvenate and heal, but always reminds us of what we have been through. This is a great metaphor for life.

In the previous chapters I spoke about some of the emotional scar tissue I've collected in my life, and there will be more of that to come, but for now I'd like to take some time to look at the physical stuff. I have many examples of my body being completely uncooperative and my disability creating some challenging situations, and people often judge me based solely on their perception of my physical ability. Often I'm met with questions that float across people's eyes but dare not pass their lips. This is where I'm going to try to address all things medical, and hopefully clarify some of these things.

I've never thought that I spend that much time thinking about medical stuff, but when I reflected more specifically on all of my experiences and all of the drama, I realised that it's actually a fairly prominent aspect of my life. My disability has always just been a part of my life as well as my family's lives, so whenever I went to a doctor or had a surgery, it never really clicked in my mind as "a medical moment". It wasn't compartmentalised in that way, it was just a moment in our lives where we needed to do something medically related.

ACCIDENT-PRONE BUT NOT FRAGILE

Having a disability doesn't necessarily mean that you're not healthy. I'm not sick, my body is just highly uncooperative and regularly has its own agenda. This is a common misconception that we need to fight. If people keep thinking that all disabled people are automatically sick and always have a problem of some kind, we're not going to be able to move to a place where people with disabilities are treated as the capable people that we are.

It may seem as though I'm undermining this idea with the stories that follow, but remember this is a condensed timeline. These experiences have been collected (like an expensive coin collection) over the past two-and-a-half decades.

I've been quite lucky in my life because my disability hasn't had too many drastic effects on my health. Maybe it's just in the way we have approached my disability – it's not the focus of most conversations we have. We've never boxed my disability into a purely "medical" category because it affects so many other aspects of our lives. All of them, actually.

Life has a certain level of risk. This doesn't change when you have a disability. Obviously, depending on your disability, there are different things that need more attention, but you can still have experiences.

I have always been very accident-prone and I thought I'd share some of my stories with you. Most of, if not all, my accidents or injuries have involved my wheelchair or my disability in some way. I've dislocated fingers and caught my toes on table legs when my foot has been hanging off the edge of my wheelchair while moving at speed to get somewhere. I've sprained my ankles countless times. I sprained my elbow when I fell sideways into an empty flower bed at school (I misjudged the distance because I was expecting to see flowers and I had always been able to gauge the distance based on the flowers, but they had been removed) and my wheelchair landed on top of my arm. It was reminiscent of my fourth birthday party, when I landed upside down on the roses. These were pretty minor incidents, though, with no serious injuries.

I've had some worse experiences, but they've led to some decent stories. Just a few examples for your entertainment...

I fractured my heel once. A collection of random things led to this. I was in our lounge, lying on a mattress on the floor. We were going to be giving a presentation for a Scouts event at St George's Cathedral and Mom was getting me dressed. As she put on my pants, she went to move me onto the couch, but when she grabbed my leg (in typical Mom style) my foot fell to the floor and my heel hit the floor from about a metre up. We didn't make too much of it because that kind of thing happens all the time; my body doesn't act in expected ways. But when we arrived at the event, my foot was so painful and swollen that I couldn't put a shoe on it. As I got out of the car and into my wheelchair, the pain was so intense that I wasn't able to speak. Luckily for me, it was a Scouts event and their mantra of "be prepared" was helpful in that moment. One of the leaders who had organised our attendance got some painkillers from the first-aid kit. The only problem was that it was a capsule, which I can't swallow (it's a disability thing), and we had to figure something out. So there we were, sitting at the back of the church, opening the capsule, and I proceeded to lick the powder off Mom's hand. I looked like I was doing drugs and I can imagine the thoughts going through all the minds of the people watching this story unfold. It took forever for my heel to heal, but on the bright side I don't walk, so I didn't have to adjust anything in my life to accommodate the healing process. I just didn't wear a shoe on that foot while it healed.

When I was 11 years old I had an experience with my wheelchair that changed how I related to it. I was at home with my personal-care assistant and Mom was on her way home to fetch me for an appointment with the surgeon to discuss my last hamstring transfer surgery. When Mom arrived we ran to the gate, but we hadn't put my seat belt on. Normally that wouldn't be a problem, but on this day my wheelchair decided to teach us a life lesson. While we were running, my seat belt (that's supposed to keep me safe – yes, I can appreciate the irony!) got caught in the push rim of the wheelchair, and the chair stopped, swiftly. I did not. The forward momentum of the running and sudden stopping sent me flying forwards towards the ground like a baby bird that's fallen out of its nest and is attempting to fly for the first time. At that stage I had minimal protective reflexes and couldn't put my arms up to stop myself in a fall. So naturally, I fell on my face. Chin first. Then teeth. When my face hit the rugged bricks I was in shock, and took a few seconds to process what had just happened. I thought that I had lost all of my front teeth and when I was picked up off the floor I frantically scanned to see where they were. There was blood everywhere and I didn't know where it was coming from. Upon closer inspection, we discovered I had a decent cut on my chin – the first point of connection between my face and the floor – and my teeth were still in my mouth, but they were loose for weeks. They were ground down about 5mm straight across, which is arguably a good outcome, considering the alternative.

Since we were already going to the hospital, it made sense to stick to the plan – there would just be a bit more work for my surgeon than he was expecting. Before looking at my legs, he quickly had to fix my face. I remember sitting in his waiting room, still bleeding, for what was probably just a minute but felt like forever, across from an elderly man who was very openly unimpressed with the entire situation. He looked at me crying and bleeding, and, with a huge indignant sigh, said, "Ugh, children." We were handling a slight crisis, so the least he could have done was to show some compassion. Anyway, everything got sorted out (I didn't need stitches, which I was happy about) and we carried on with our lives, with a mandate to eat soft things like soup, jelly and custard until my gums regained their grip on my teeth. Doctor's orders.

The last memory I'll share here happened in my first year at university. We had booked a midmorning appointment to apply for a Schengen visa because we were going to the Netherlands to do some work with the KidsRights Foundation. I had classes all day, starting at 8am, so the plan was for me to go to my first class, and Mom would fetch me for the appointment and then drop me back at campus in time for my afternoon classes. Everything was going according to plan. (I feel this is the time you should start questioning the plan – it was too simple.) Mom arrived to pick me up. It was raining, so she parked outside my lecture venue so I wouldn't have to walk in the rain and get too wet. She was early, so she decided to get the ramp out before I got there to save time. When my class ended I made my way to the back of the car to stay as dry as possible, as was standard procedure. The plan was that Mom would then carry me to the front seat, just as we had done hundreds of times before. Mom lifted me out of my wheelchair and walked towards the open front car door – and tripped over the edge of the already-set-up ramp, and we fell onto the tarmac. I landed quite solidly on the bottom of my back and Mom landed on top of me, but her mama bear instincts kicked in and she braced with her knee so it wouldn't be that bad. Before we could even call for help, there was a group of about 15 students ready to get involved and help us. It was a good thing it happened during the 15 minutes when classes were changing, otherwise we might still have been there...

It was amazing to have so many people willing to help us and make sure we were fine. I don't fully know how everything came together, but somebody picked me up and put me into the car and went back to make sure Mom was all right. They didn't realise I didn't have the balance to keep myself in the car, so I nearly fell out of it. Luckily Mom was paying attention and shouted for someone to put my seat belt on so that I would be 100% safe. My back was a bit stuffed and Mom's knee was quite bruised and cut up. I must say, though, that was one of the fastest and smoothest visa applications I've ever experienced. I think they recognised the state we were in and I'm sure they wanted to get us out of there. When I got back to campus we couldn't get ice packs and settled for strategically placed cold Cokes, which worked pretty well. I do think my current back issues may stem from this incident...

These stories are a tad ridiculous, and while my experiences may not have been enjoyable at the time, I'm glad I have stories to share. My disability didn't take experiences from me; it has contributed to me having some more great stories to tell.

WHO'S THE BOSS?

We already know that my body and disability are a rock-solid rebellious pair prone to public spectacle and scene-making. Even still, there are moments when I accept that my body can take the lead and make some decisions. I don't love it (that's all about me enjoying being in control), but sometimes it's good to listen to what your body is telling you.

[TANGENT]
To fully understand why this is extra hard for me, you need to understand how our family tends to deal with medical crises.

My family functions with a sort of counterintuitive hypochondria. What does this even mean? We're definitely not hypochondriacs. And we're definitely not ostriches with our heads stuck in the sand. If anything, we underreact, thinking we have a minor problem that turns out to be quite a big deal. I once thought I was just having really hectic period cramps, when I actually had a bowel obstruction and ended up in hospital for four days. Dad had "indigestion" for a while, but it turned out he was actually having a series of mini heart attacks. That is a pretty radical example, but don't worry, he is all good now.

My family's go-to strategy generally works like this: something comes up, we make a plan and find a way to move forwards. We don't go to the doctor at the first sign of a cough. We have to be fully woman – or man – down for an extended period of time for an illness to be taken seriously. I've struggled with allergies basically my whole life and only addressed the issue in my first year of university. I was pretty sure I needed glasses from my first year at university but only went to get them seven years later. There were just more pressing things going on in my life that were prioritised. Don't look at us like that – you know we're not the only people who do this!
[TANGENT OVER]

Living with disability can be a lot to handle. It's definitely a marathon, as it is something that is going to be with me for the rest of my life. The physical aspects of my disability are manageable – we've found strategies that work for me – but more often than not it's the stigma (like an uninvited guest who everyone awkwardly avoids) accompanying it that makes it more difficult to keep motivated throughout the marathon. I have to prove myself to people in almost every situation in which I find myself. Although there are people who are constantly fighting and working to dismantle the stigma around disability, and progress has been made for sure, this is still the current reality. In a medical context, this stigma is definitely alive and well, and I will get into this in a minute.

I think a massive barrier for accessing different solutions is assumptions, especially in medical spaces. In many of my interactions with medical professionals, I haven't always been taken seriously when it comes to understanding my body and what works (and what doesn't work) for me. Many times I've said something and it's been disregarded, and yet it's been acted on when someone non-disabled, like Mom, has said the same thing. Or I've asked a question about a medication in a drip and been told that I didn't need to worry about it... The thing is, it's my body, so you should be answering my questions instead of brushing them off. Once I insisted that the nurse give me the information and she did, I was happy. Involve me in my care, people.

Medical procedures (like surgeries, bowel programmes/management systems and so on) are a part of disabled life. It is how we manage our bodies in order to live life. However, every disabled person has a unique relationship with their body and how they manage aspects of their disability as a part of (often) everyday life is unique to their circumstances. This part of disability is the piece of the puzzle that remains most in the shadows and many people don't talk about it because it's deemed impolite or private. Some disabled people prefer to keep these things private; I choose to share details like these as a way to raise awareness. Each approach is acceptable – it obviously just comes down to what works for each individual.

I have had various surgeries on my legs since the age of two. I had surgery for my Achilles tendons twice, hamstring transfers twice and an adductor release once, which felt like the worst one to me because I had full leg casts on both legs, with a stick in between to keep my legs open. (This was seen and used as an additional, conveniently placed carrying aid.) I've also had a few stints of Botox in my legs and hands – it's not only for sorting out wrinkles and crow's feet! In my layperson understanding, it essentially paralyses the muscle it is injected into, so it relaxes overactive muscles (which is where spasms come from), and you can then work with it through physio and more to achieve your desired function level. The thing with this is that it isn't guaranteed to work – sometimes it worked and other times it didn't. Sometimes you have to roll the dice and then work with what happens. I started having issues with my knees halfway through high school. My kneecaps were migrating up because of the stiffness in my legs, and so I had surgery to move them down again. These operations were done separately, and the purpose was purely pain management. Remember the drama around this during my first week at university? This was the surgery.

None of these operations really bothered me, in that I wasn't stressed or nervous about them. It was kind of just a thing we did every couple of years and after they did the operations I had casts for six weeks and got to draw all over my legs without getting into trouble. Obviously, there were times I wasn't happy about having the casts, but when you're little, it's related to the simple things. Like when it gets itchy and you can't reach it (not that that wasn't something I was used to dealing with anyway) or when it's a really nice, sunny day and everyone else is swimming and you can't.

My last surgery of this kind was a second hamstring transfer when I was 12 years old. This was done to make walking (assisted) easier – I was still walking a bit at that point, but not to an extent that was functionally meaningful. It was right around this time that I started asserting more authority over what was happening with my body.

It's important to see where the journey of working with your body goes, and evolving when you need to. Ideas change, and what matters most to you changes too. I appreciate that I was given the space to be my own ship's captain, which is not always the case for a lot of people with disabilities. There are many things we don't have control over, and often one of these is our body, but there should always be options available. One of the lessons that has been instilled in me is that regardless of the situation or challenge, there are always options. The thing that is always good to remember is that when you are treating a disability, it exists within a person. That person has feelings and opinions about what is happening with and to their bodies and their disabilities, and these can evolve, so we all need to be open to hear and embrace the evolution.

There are so many things in my life that I used to accept as being "the way it is" and just part of my life, in particular the way my body functions (or fails to function). Certain foods don't work for me because of tactile aversion because of my CP, and I've always said I don't like them. (Sometimes that's an easier explanation than going with the "it's because of my disability" route.) I dealt with my body's idiosyncrasies on an emotional level at an early age, so they didn't impact my self-esteem in any serious way.

As I got older, though, I reached a point where certain things, like bladder incontinence and bowel issues, became less acceptable to me. I was tired of having so little control over my body and constantly living on the edge. I've never had great balancing skills and I eventually went on a mission, investigating potential alternatives.

This is the part of my story where I feel I hold the most unexpressed frustration because it's hardly ever appropriate to discuss bladder (over)activity and bowel movements. I know that many of my stories focus on this topic, but it's a big deal. Non-disabled people may not see it as such because it's second nature and automatic for them, so it doesn't take up so much space in their lives. Here, I hope to share a potentially new perspective. Whenever I'm speaking to other people with physical disabilities, regardless of how they've gained their disability, these issues seem to be common ground, and inevitably come up at some point in the conversation. To me, it shows that it's an important thing to discuss and get comfortable with, and to find (and share) solutions. There are probably a few people who believe it's not appropriate to discuss these things here either, but this is my story, so...

My unique brand of CP includes lifelong bladder incontinence. I never quite managed to get a handle on potty training. We only discovered incontinence pads when I was about nine years old, after trying regular sanitary pads and finding them unsuccessful. There definitely needs to be more variety and options in this area. People come in all shapes and sizes, with their own preferences. I've found that generally, the size options begin at medium. (I don't know why this happens and I don't know who was consulted on this decision, but I definitely have some questions and suggestions...) It's also difficult to find incontinence pads that still make you feel sexy and dignified. I don't think they've been designed with this purpose in mind. If you are a small person you either need to get giant ones with much too much material or you have to get kiddies' versions and choose between *Paw Patrol* and *Dora the Explorer*.

Also included in my CP cocktail is the added bonus of chronic constipation (such a joy). By trying to solve my bladder issue through medication, it antagonised the bowel issues. Mom always said this combination made me "a cement mixer". I think this is a hilarious and accurate analogy.

I was never really too concerned about (or committed to) managing this area of my life. In my mind, I was busy living and I didn't have the time or energy to deal with it. So, for the first 17 years of my life we generally just went with the flow (excuse the pun) and whatever happened, happened. When it comes to my bowel function, my body only really works when I tell it to. This is probably not the most medically sound strategy (definitely not), but it's what we did and it was the life strategy that worked for me. When I was 17, we were introduced to the concept of colonic irrigations. These are basically intense enemas where you pump litres of water into your body, and gravity gets involved and the world falls out of your bum. Super glamorous. I have heard that a number of celebrities have had these done, though, so there's that. We did this for a year or so until a nursing friend mentioned that you can get home irrigation kits. Life-changing.

[TANGENT]
Here's something that really gets under my skin... I feel there is so much focus on what diagnosis someone has and it limits how we access solutions. I believe that there has to be more creativity around solution-finding – focusing on what the challenges are instead of taking a diagnosis at face value. There are similar challenges for people who have different diagnoses, like bowel management being a common challenge for various disabilities, but the solutions offered (at least in my experience) are largely curtailed by the label of your disability. Colonic irrigation is a standard go-to management strategy for spina bifida, for example, and even though the challenge is similar for CP, we weren't told about it for decades. We found out about it through a chance meeting with another woman in a wheelchair who did it and shared contact details of her person.
[TANGENT OVER]

I don't want my body to be the sole dictator of the direction of my life. This is an overarching idea in my life and is also true for how I spend the hours in my day. In this case, I'm not going to take a tablet (because these don't really work for me) and wait hours for them to work their way through my system. I think I'm just much too impatient for this strategy. I'm very much on board with instant gratification, hence colonic irrigation. Everybody is different and I fully believe you have to do what works for you – for all aspects of your life.

I'm still not convinced that having a completely clean colon is a key life priority. Here's my logic... Typically, it's seen as a good thing to be "regular". I think that works well when you can take yourself to a toilet, and when nature calls you can just get up and go. Considering that I don't have that option, and remembering my body's spiteful tendencies, when I hear "regular" I'm thinking that's a really risky, unpredictable and unreliable strategy for my life. I'm thinking that it can then happen at any time, and then I'll be having anxiety about the Russian roulette going on in my body. It's far more reliable to take a couple of hours to irrigate once a week and know for sure (because we're not telling my body to activate) that I'm not going to poop in my pants for the next six days. Life is all about balancing different choices and consequences, and my disability means there are a few additional things to consider. Yes, patience definitely has a place in my life, but that place is not a bathroom.

I am, however, convinced that the bladder is, in fact, the true boss of the body, at least for me, and it has been in control for far too long. I always just figured that my life would be that way forever. That I would never be able to drink more than half a glass of anything and still be able to sit in my friend's car without leaving a wet seat behind me when they put me back in my wheelchair and we got wherever we were going. That if I was wet, I would just have to stay that way until I got home. That I would never be able to wear cute underwear because incontinence pads are not designed to be cute, they're designed to be functional. Mostly. I can't talk about this for too long, otherwise it will definitely turn into a rant. I didn't think of these things as barriers per se, more like a part of the deal; something the people in my life need to get used to and wrap their heads around, just as I had to. If they couldn't, that was okay. How could I expect them to deal with these things? That's too intense for a friendship to withstand. And I don't want to be that needy friend, the one everyone else has to make plans around. Years later, I have realised that this is the wrong attitude (see how internalised ableism sneaks into my thoughts and actions when I'm not looking?) and that that is actually exactly what friendships are for.

I have found people who combat all of my overthinking about my body and its random outbursts and power struggles – people who don't make a big deal when they need to put a towel down on a seat; who don't point it out when I suddenly disappear and on my return am wearing a completely new outfit because the one I was wearing was wet. I don't know how to explain what these small moments of peace mean to me. They are a recognition of empowerment, and they're just as important as any of the big things. These moments make the "embarrassing" experiences much more bearable.

Taking control

Are you ready for another important and confusing conversation? We've discussed the indisputable fact that my disability leaves me needing significant assistance in many areas of my life. Where this gets confusing is that even though I need all of this help, I don't feel as though I am unable to live a life with independence. I think it's because my disability has taught me a different definition of what it means to be independent. There's so much pressure to do things in a mainstream way and that's often seen as "independence", so when I'm eating popcorn (or anything) like a chameleon – sticking my tongue out and licking it to get it into my mouth – people think it's weird and their eyes ask why nobody is helping me. This perpetuates the pressure to conform to those norms, and embraces the idea that if I can't do things in the standard, non-disabled way, I should be helped.

To me, it's not about doing things completely on my own, it's an attitude. It's recognising that the people in my life can assist me to a point of independence. Trying to do things completely independently has its obvious benefits, like being able to do stuff without other people, but I also think it could be an incredibly lonely experience, and in my situation I can't do a lot, which can be frustrating. I don't want to deal with the frustrations of not being able to do all of those things and have that lead to a negative relationship with my disability. I would much rather acknowledge the things I need help with, and be supported with things I'm not so great with.

This is an ongoing journey of discovery and it's impacted by so many things. I'm grateful that I've been disabled for my whole life and have got used to people watching me and being curious about what I'm doing. I'm not self-conscious about people paying attention to my unique strategies of getting things done. I do sometimes have to check myself and stop the internalised ableism that happens when questions seep into my headspace and I overthink them. This happens mostly when I'm meeting new people and I'm alone with them, like in a meeting or on a date. I need to remind myself that the fact that I need help to eat or use a bathroom is a normal thing; it's a part of life. I have to have the internal conversation that it is possible for people not to have issues with being helpful and I should be making space for that possibility.

I do enjoy being able to do things on my own, though. There are many instances where I'm able to act independently (in the mainstream understanding). For example, if I am working on my laptop and I have everything I need within arm's reach, I can function on my own without assistance for hours on end. But this has never really extended to my body. Most activities that involve my body will involve other people, and "simple" things like going to the bathroom have definitely never been on the independent activity list.

It became more important to me to have more control over my body and its fundamental functions when I started university and was invited to do active and adventurous things (like the Cape Town Cycle Tour) and I needed to find solutions that would work when spending hours out on the road, without access to proper toilets or bathrooms. I got on board when I realised that the go-with-the-flow strategy doesn't really work for such situations. And remember, the ability to hold it in was just not something I could do at that point.

Life has interesting ways of making you look at situations with different perspectives and think about things in a new light.

I had always been very opposed to using catheters because I had only used one once before when I was about six years old, and that was a traumatic experience for me. But when the opportunity arose to do the Cycle Tour, I wanted to do the race more than I was scared of, or averse to, using the catheter. The benefits outweighed the negatives. I realised that once the catheter is in my body (as I mentioned earlier, we use indwelling catheters for adventurous missions – this means it stays in my body for an extended period and my bladder can empty constantly) and is properly secured, it is a more dignified solution. It was far less of a personal thing to ask someone to empty a bag attached to my leg, and it had the added bonus of allowing me to drink as much as I wanted without worrying about my bladder overflowing and creating a scene. So having eased up on my anti-catheter position, it was easier to look at different options that I hadn't been open to previously.

GETTING TO THE BOTTOM OF THINGS

For literally years I have struggled with constant bladder infections – every couple of months I would have another one. (Cranberry juice was a good friend of mine.) It became especially problematic in my last year of undergrad and my honours year. The rate at which I was going through outfits in a day was becoming particularly ridiculous. I think my pain threshold is fairly high and I got used to it, so I didn't think they were that bad. You know it's a problem when you know the names of all the different antibiotics... This, combined with the new adventure strategy, had us thinking more about what would work best for me when I start working. I needed a solution that allowed me to be more independent in my bladder control and management plans.

After going to the doctor for what felt like the billionth bladder infection I was referred to a urologist, Larry Jee, so that we could figure out what was happening and regain a level of control of the situation. I think his name is cool – it sounds badass to me. I went into the consultation with a semi-open mind, but also a very clear objective – more independence. If he suggested something that didn't fit well with this objective, then it wasn't an option. We gave my history and all the relevant information for a brainstorming session to find viable solutions.

While we were having this conversation I remembered that during a previous hospital stay they had done an ultrasound and found a bladder stone. The doctor told us not to worry about it because it was too big to pass and it wasn't an immediate problem. (This just shows how different things are important to different people.) It made sense to me because at the time they were working to identify what was making me sick, and it wasn't my bladder. Mentioning this issue (as a throwaway comment) to Larry changed the entire discussion because now there was a possible explanation for why my bladder was being so erratic. Larry is great because he only gives options if he knows they're viable; he doesn't suggest things that aren't attainable with my body. Now, the plan had to change.

To start with, we needed to sort out the bladder stone before we made any other plans because this could be the root of many of my problems. So I was scheduled for bladder stone surgery. I don't remember the technical name for this. I do remember someone in my family making a joke that I was going to get "de-pitted", like an olive or something. I appreciated the joke.

This was the first step towards bladder independence, so I was weirdly excited. The procedure took longer than expected because the stone was much bigger than expected. I mean, it was already big (2cm in diameter, according to the most recent ultrasound), but when they went in to get it, we're told that it was at least the size of a golf ball, probably bigger. We were also told that it had probably been growing for a couple of years. That's ridiculous. I wanted to be able to say "Oh, it must have started here..." There's no way of knowing when it started, but I just decided that if it had been there for two years, then it *must* have started out as a Kilimanjaro dust speck. That idea is probably largely inaccurate, but I liked the idea of having a piece of an incredible, powerful mountain inside of me. Is that weird?

We got the stone. I had signed that form that allows the hospital to dispose of the stone as medical waste, because I don't want to see it or keep it. Clearly someone missed that directive because when I woke up there it was in a jar next to me on my pillow. Gross. (Just to be clear, it doesn't come out of my body as a giant stone, although that would be cool. It comes out as a whole bunch of teeny-tiny stones.) I had to stay in hospital overnight for them to flush my bladder properly, to try to prevent bladder stones from re-forming. Apparently, once you get one stone they tend to recur. So that's great. I have had a few after this too (I grow them like a champion), but it seems we have everything under control for now.

Before we knew what was happening with my bladder I was having horrendous nausea. All day. Every day. I think nausea is one of the worst forms of sickness because it lingers like a fog and you can't get away from it. To make things worse, because I spend my days in a wheelchair I can't really try different positions to alleviate it. I was prescribed some pretty intense medication that works in seconds, but the nausea would inevitably come back. I guess I just learnt how to function with it. So, when I woke up after the procedure and my first thought wasn't "Ugh, I'm nauseous", it was an amazing feeling. I know there are bigger things in my life than being nausea-free, but I'd lived with feeling nauseous for so long that I didn't realise it wasn't normal to feel as though you're going to get sick every day. I knew that we were on the road to independence and I was excited about that.

Within a few weeks I had recovered and we moved on to the next step of this journey – tests. We did a urodynamics test, which assesses a whole lot of things like bladder capacity, leakage, and your ability to hold and keep your bladder full, and your bladder's behaviour is monitored throughout. For some reason I had never thought about being able to test these things, never mind manage them. It took a while to get this test done because I was still fighting bladder infections fairly regularly (my bladder was learning how to live without the stone, and it took a second to normalise), so we had to wait for a relatively healthy period so as not to affect the findings of the test. We got a lot of helpful information from this test. My bladder capacity was something ridiculous like 180ml. (The normal bladder capacity of an adult is between about 300ml and 400ml.) I mean, it's no wonder I was always leaking and never dry!

Even just having that information made it easier to manage my bladder. As I now knew I had a minuscule capacity, sharing drinks became a thing we did more often so I didn't reach a point of overflow.

MY MITROFANOFF

When my bladder had sufficiently got over itself, I went back to Larry to work out the next steps. We spoke about intermittent catheterisation, which would solve the problem of constantly being wet, but with my limited dexterity it wouldn't solve the independence problem. After discussing the various options we had at our disposal, Larry suggested that we could use my appendix. I was so confused, but I didn't ask any follow-up questions about it, which is very unlike me. But when we got home I researched "bladder + appendix procedures" and there it was. The Mitrofanoff!

Basically, the Mitrofanoff is a procedure where the appendix (or in some cases a small section of the intestine) is used as a conduit between the bladder and the abdomen, so you can catheterise through your abdomen instead of down below. In my case we used my appendix. Ideally, the stoma (this is an artificial opening) is made in the belly button for aesthetic purposes because it's less visible and more accessible. This was the plan for mine too.

[TANGENT]
A week before the surgery I had a scan to check the size of my appendix and to ensure it was long enough to attach to my bladder and reach my abdomen. I didn't realise how stressed I was about this (and how I hadn't thought about how problematic it would be if there was an issue with my appendix) until I was inside that machine, having the scan. All I was thinking throughout the scan was "Please, I need my body to work with me right now". If it wasn't big enough, I wouldn't be able to have this life-changing surgery and we'd have to go back to the drawing board. That would have been a tough one to process. They did the scan and couldn't see my appendix. Are you serious? Body, we spoke about this! I started spiralling, thinking that maybe I was one of those people born without one because they say the appendix doesn't serve a purpose. (You know, evolution and things...) Typical that just when we had found a purpose and a use for this organ, we'd find out I didn't have one. I was stressed and overthinking my life without an appendix for a few days because they'd scheduled me for a second scan. They assured me that there was no reason to assume it wasn't there, and that it's just sneaky and likes to hide behind other organs.

After the second scan there was nothing to worry about. It was present and big enough. (It was on the smaller side, but workable.) Big sigh of relief from my side.

[TANGENT OVER]

My surgery was scheduled for the end of July 2017. I was really excited and focused on how it could change my life. I now had to wait a few months for the surgery day to arrive. Having surgery has never been that stressful for me, mostly because all of my previous surgeries were on my legs and I had rationalised that if something went wrong it wouldn't be too bad because I don't really use my legs to function in my everyday life. This one was different – they were reorganising and repurposing my organs. It was high stakes.

As luck would have it, the day of my surgery was a logistically complex day. Dad took me to the hospital to get checked in and sort out all of the medical aid admin. Mom had to be somewhere for a few hours in the morning and would be at the hospital before I went in for the surgery. That all worked out as we'd intended.

The first few hours were taken up with the usual pre-op prep. When the anaesthetist came in to see me, she checked my heart rate and it was apparently a bit higher than she would have liked, and she asked me, "Is your heart rate usually this high?" I have no idea what it normally is, but I also don't walk around constantly checking my heart rate. She suggested I get something to keep me calm before the surgery and I told her that I wasn't able to swallow pills and she responded with, "We'll make a plan." I understood that to mean they would find an alternative to pills (like a syrup or an injection). A few minutes later a nurse arrived with a glass of water, pills and a spoon, and I realised that *this* was the version of making a plan we were working with. Just as I was debating with the nurse whether this strategy was likely to work, Mom arrived. She continued debating the point with the nurse, but we were told that alternatives weren't possible because there wasn't enough time to organise the other options.

I decided to back my body and give the tablets a go. These were crushed and placed in the spoon with some water, but it didn't change into a paste, it just stayed as grainy bits of tablet, which doesn't play nicely with my tactile aversion. It probably would have been fine, but then I coughed and aspirated the water and the calming meds. I ended up having a coughing fit and the porters arrived to take me through to pre-op a few minutes later. If I hadn't been feeling stressed before, I was then. This was followed by the nurses asking Mom to sign the permission forms before I got wheeled away. I was 23 years old. It turned this into a learning moment because the head nurse confronted them pretty sternly about their ableism in assuming that I couldn't sign for myself, even though I was of legal age. This type of thing happens all the time, but it's not that often that we find someone else calling people out before we get the chance to. It was funny, though, because after she had made this whole scene, I was coughing so much and didn't have the energy to sign, so I asked Mom to do it for me. (If I'm the one asking someone to sign on my behalf, that's totally fine... Autonomy, remember.) Seven minutes later I was rolled in and the anaesthetist was doing her thing. Anaesthetists always make me feel like a rock star just for breathing or counting backwards from 10.

The surgery took five hours or so and when I woke up I was taken to the High Care unit, where I stayed for a couple of days until the epidural was taken out. A few minutes after I woke up I was completely overwhelmed and emotional, with random outbursts of crying (it's my usual reaction to the anaesthetic), and Mom comforted me, saying everything was okay. I had just had my whole abdomen cut open and my organs rearranged, so there was a fair amount of confusion going on in my body. I was on some pretty great drugs to keep the pain at bay, so I was also a bit loopy. Because of the epidural and my meds cocktail I was relatively comfortable, but the thing that was bothering me was that I had the most intense shoulder pain. I'm told that can happen with abdominal surgeries because air gets into your body and there isn't a lot they can do about it. It simply has to work itself out.

My first full day in High Care was pretty uneventful. Some friends and family came to visit, but hospitals can be very monotonous, so you live for visiting hours. My friends James and Jess came through, and although I don't remember what we spoke about at all, apparently I said some hilarious things because of the meds. I'm told there is photo and voice note evidence of my take on reality while on "the good meds", as I called them.

I wasn't in love with having the epidural because the idea of having something sticking into my spine freaks me out. That was until I woke up at 2am in excruciating pain – the magical meds that were in the epidural had run out. The nurses were in the process of refilling it, but they hadn't yet. I was hysterical. Luckily, we had shared the important information that if I'm crying, you shouldn't ask me what's wrong, as I won't be able to respond with words. You have to ask yes/no questions because then I can respond with the appropriate nod. It's also important to make educated guesses about which questions you ask, as we don't want to waste anyone's time. The nurses were on top of this situation, so they didn't need to ask what was happening. I started appreciating the epidural and its purpose after that because the meds started flowing again and my body returned to an acceptable level of pain.

[TANGENT]
High Care is loud, with all the machines beeping to different rhythms, and not at all harmoniously. So it's hard to sleep, but I did what I could. I was happy that there was a nurse assigned specifically to me (and one other person), sitting at the foot of my bed so she could see immediately if I needed anything.

When Erin had come to visit earlier she had brought Ferrero Rocher chocolates and I was looking forward to eating them when I had the energy. She put them in the cupboard next to my bed and I could ask a nurse to get one for me when I felt like one. I woke up a while after my epidural was sorted and I just couldn't sleep. I was lying half on my back just chilling, but with no energy to make any sort of noise. Nothing interesting was happening and I was trying to drown out the beeping. A nurse came over and checked my machines ... and then she went to my cupboard. Now I was paying attention. She opened the cupboard and took out two chocolates and sat down to eat them. She then got up to leave. I was looking at her and as she walked past me she said, "Good morning!" with much more enthusiasm than was warranted at 2am.

I went back to sleep because I didn't have the energy to make a scene. When I woke up later that morning, Mom arrived with Erin and they asked me if I wanted any chocolates. We took the box out of the cupboard and there were only three left! So somebody had enjoyed themselves, and it certainly wasn't me.
[TANGENT OVER]

I like having information so that I can process all the options, potential outcomes and strategies. However, that doesn't extend to every single detail of a surgery. There, you can give me broad brushstrokes and intended outcomes and I'm fine. I don't know why this is the case, but I feel it's a good balance. I have learnt that sometimes it's okay not to see everything. Before I left High Care the nurses had to change my dressing and I wanted to see what my wound looked like and how I was healing. They told me I shouldn't look at it because in the beginning it always looks worse than it is. They were right – it didn't look great. I wasn't prepared for the gauze, drains and catheter pipes around and in my body. After seeing my abdomen and hearing from the nurses that my scar was looking beautiful, I decided I didn't need to be involved or engaged in this process next time.

I spent two days in High Care and as the epidural wore off once it was taken out, my big takeaway was to never underestimate the power of a Voltaren suppository. Seriously though, even though it's less than dignified and pleasant, these made me so happy and took away most of my pain in minutes. Don't judge it until you try it.

Looking back at my nine-day hospital stay, I was grumpy (for various reasons) for most of my time there. I feel a smidgen bad about this, but it was how I felt at the time and there was a lot going on in my body that I was temporarily unhappy about.

With a big surgery like this one, I understand one concern is circulation. I have bad circulation at the best of times (perks of being a wheelchair user), so it's fair to assume it could be problematic. To alleviate some risk here, I had electric compression socks. I thought they were cool for the first few days because I'd never used them before. I'm a relatively tiny adult human, so I had to use the paediatric version of the socks to ensure they would fit and serve their purpose. I wore them all day, so when they were removed a few days in, I didn't want them any more. We stopped using these on day four.

Ahead of being taken to the general ward, where I'd be living for the next week, I had to be moved to a different bed. (Apparently beds are specifically assigned to each ward or unit and they can't be moved out of them.) It was an intense moment in my recovery and I had to practise some heavy breathing as they quickly and efficiently lifted me, along with all the recovery paraphernalia, onto my new bed. Once I was comfortably settled in my new bed I was moved to the general ward and I felt good about it. It was progress. I lay down for the first three days, unable to laugh or sneeze or anything that required stomach muscles in any form. I was bleak that the core I'd been working on for years was gone in a matter of hours. I never knew how much a person uses these muscles for basically every movement, even the tiniest ones. Am I happy with the outcome and was it a worthwhile sacrifice of my abs? One hundred percent, yes.

Hospitals can be incredibly boring places, so someone coming to visit was always a breath of fresh air and a much-needed break from the monotony. My first morning in the general ward was just about settling in to this new space, meeting the new nurses and getting comfy. I was embracing the idea of just lying in my new bed, doing nothing except healing. A few hours later, a physio walked into the room and made her way towards me. I was confused... Why was she coming to me? Somewhere in my subconscious I knew that a key factor in recovering from abdominal surgery is getting up, out of bed, and mobile. I figured that I was exempt from that requirement since I'm a wheelchair user and don't walk anywhere, ever. Not the case. She came in with enthusiasm and told me I was going to work on sitting up in the bed, and then we would maybe try to get me sitting in my wheelchair for a bit. The physio, Caryn, looked familiar to me and once we started chatting I found out that we actually knew each other – Mom had taught her in Grade 7 and coached her in hockey. It's amazing to see how people reconnect in the most random, unexpected of places.

The purpose of doing the physio in the hospital was twofold. First, it was about getting mobile, and second it was for chest physio. I was sceptical about the reason for this because I had never had any significant issues in this area, so why were we starting now? About 10 minutes into the chest physio portion of the session I felt the purpose. I was coughing so much with so much phlegm that I didn't even know was there. This was possibly a result of my aspirating the calming meds. Okay, fine, maybe they know what they're doing when they prescribe things. Let's be honest, I wouldn't be me if I didn't question everything that's going on.

That session was a lot for me. We had to take it easy and decided we would try getting me into my wheelchair the next day. I was nervous about that, which was a weird feeling for me because my chair has always been a positive thing in my life, but in that moment it was scary. I felt stressed that if I sat fully upright (which I would be doing in my wheelchair) I would "fall out of myself". If you've ever had surgery like this I hope this is a relatable fear. With some convincing from Caryn that I would not have my internal organs splattered all over the hospital room floor, we moved me into my wheelchair. I made it. As this was going down, Warren – who was by now my brother-in-law – walked into the room with hot chocolate. That made me happy. This lasted 30 minutes or so until I felt nauseous and went pale, and needed to get back in the bed.

Each day I was able to spend more and more time in my wheelchair, and I was eventually allowed to leave the room. I was so excited! I could go and eat with people in the restaurant downstairs, and I also got to move to the window side of the room, so that made the days more interesting. It's in the small things.

Let me give you a full picture of what my body was dealing with. I had the usual IV drip for medication and hydration; a drain in my left side with a bag to collect the gunk inside; and a suprapubic catheter on my lower right side, just above my pubic bone. My incision was covered by gauze and dressing, and the stoma had a catheter in it to keep it open while it healed.

In my High Care pain management haze I registered something that simultaneously confused me and made me think I had a really smart medical team working with me. The IV was in my right arm, but there was another one in my left hand. When I asked what that was for, they told me it was there in case the other one stopped working, as they could then easily just switch over. That blew my mind. Genius. It's virtually impossible to get my veins to cooperate when it comes to inserting an IV, so having a backup plan was a smart move.

I was very aware of the drain, convinced it was going to hook on something. It never did. I was shocked and slightly disgusted when they removed it. I had questions... How could it be so long? It was as long as my body is wide, so where did it fit? I don't need the answers to this, but still. I was so much more comfortable and happy without that drain. Maybe that was the source of all my grumpiness...

Nine days after my surgery I went home to recover further. I left with the suprapubic catheter and a newly dressed scar, which also served the purpose of keeping the catheter in the stoma. After two weeks I had to return to the hospital to have everything taken out. I was looking forward to no longer having all the post-surgery stuff. It was interesting and kind of magical to see how everything worked. Larry arrived to take everything out and there was a gathering of nurses behind him because they were interested too. They'd never seen this procedure before.

The first step was removing the suprapubic catheter, which after almost four weeks of being in my body was pretty securely in there because my skin had grown a little too attached to it. This is when your ability to heal can sometimes be problematic, but they got it out. Larry cut the stitches, looked at me and said, "This is going to hurt" – and before I could even get my head around that fact, it was already out. It took my breath away and instantly made me want to vomit, but I prefer the band-aid method to taking it slowly. Then we had to wait a few minutes for my bladder to fill enough to test the stoma. As Larry explained every step of the process, it was like a magic trick and he was a magician, and we were all intrigued by each step. He put the catheter into the stoma, and after five seconds of us all holding our breath, it started flowing. It was remarkable. This was the moment that I decided I have so much faith in medical science and the things that are possible. If you can make an appendix work with a bladder, what can you not do?

There were a few things I didn't know or realise before we began this journey that should have been more obvious to me. I was under the impression that we would do the surgery and that as soon as it had healed enough and we were able to use a catheter in the stoma, it would just work and I would never leak again. It's not like flipping a switch. This is not a quick fix and I didn't realise that bladder training is a thing, and it's a process. My bladder has to learn that we work differently now and use a new route. It has taken time and much trial and error to get to a method that works for me. My management strategy now includes two types of medication (one helps with holding it in and the other reduces bladder spasms) and a phone alarm every three hours during the day to remind me to catheterise. The latter is important because before having the Mitrofanoff there was no routine when it came to how and when my bladder worked. It's slowly learning to regulate without the alarm, which is a nice new feature for my body. We've also discovered that catheters are expensive! I'm extremely grateful to have my monthly supply sponsored by the medical company Akacia Medical. It's a massive relief that we don't have to worry about this part of managing my disability. Purchasing catheters is not just about being able to wee; it's an investment in my independence. I think many of the decisions we make as disabled people are based not only on physical needs but also, very importantly, on all the emotional and social aspects of life.

[TANGENT]
Being disabled is an expensive endeavour. Just doing "normal" things often requires special equipment that you have to purchase, and it's largely consumable items that you're going to continue to need as long as you're alive. To add to this, whenever something is made or sold specifically for disabled people, the price goes up exponentially. For example, a while ago I was looking for a phone stand for my wheelchair. I found one that was hundreds of rands and when I searched for a similar one without the "wheelchair" tag, there was an almost identical product for about R80. So now I don't look for anything wheelchair-specific because it's hard to justify paying such high prices for items that are available for the mainstream with minimal impact on your wallet. We have to find creative ways to solve these challenges and I'm learning that sometimes things that are designed for particular purposes can also be used for other things, and this is where we develop disabled creativity and a different way of thinking about how things work.
[TANGENT OVER]

Getting this surgery has given me more than just the ability to control my bladder. It's enabled and empowered me to engage more fully in life. I've had my Mitrofanoff for a few years now and it has been truly life-changing. I no longer need to use incontinence pads all the time (I still use them sometimes, though, just in case) and it does make me feel more confident. I never understood how much of my headspace was being occupied by the challenges my bladder has created. And yes, I am now consciously thinking about my bladder and how to manage it more regularly, but these thoughts are logical and practical in nature – like how many catheters I need to pack in my bag for the amount of time I'm out for – instead of being anxiety-driven and making me feel as though I'm not in control of what happens.

I have worked out a strategy to catheterise myself so that I can go somewhere alone and be self-sufficient in that way, as long as I have my bag with me in an accessible place. It does get more complicated if I have multiple layers of clothing on, but we find ways. If I'm with other people I usually ask them to assist me because it takes me a long time to do it myself – I think the fastest I've done it is about nine minutes – so it's much faster and frankly, it's easier. It's not so hard for me to ask for help with it any more because it's not as intimate and personal as asking someone to take my pants off and hold me on a toilet. It's more comfortable for all of us.

As I've mentioned in earlier chapters, I will always rely on other people to a certain extent. It makes it easier when everyone understands me and we're on the same page. My hospital stay for my Mitrofanoff laid a solid foundation of understanding for future visits. We go to the same hospital, the same ward with the same nurses. It means there is much less stress for everyone because I don't have to re-explain my disability-related needs every time. In general life, too, these are the things that suck my energy. Having to tell people over and over again why something needs to change or why I need help with something is tiring.

I'm so grateful to all the medical professionals – doctors, nurses, therapists – and every other person who has gone on this medical journey with me. It's been an intense learning experience for all of us, and I know it can be overwhelming at times. It's been one of big leaps and certain high-risk moves. It's shown me just how incredible the human body is, how adaptable it is and how it gets us through the craziness of life, albeit with a few scars and stories along the way.

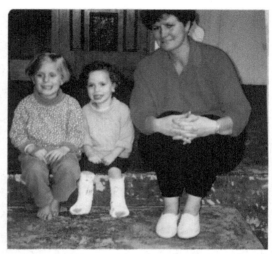

Me, aged two, with Mom and Erin after my first operation. (1996)

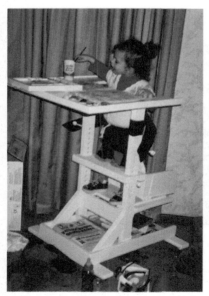

My first standing frame was amazing. I used it for nine years, which is unheard of with equipment like this, thanks to Austin Byrne's carpentry genius. (1997)

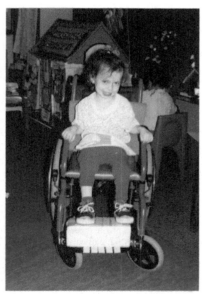

My first wheelchair was much too big for me, so we made a plan with a polystyrene block and duct tape. I was three years old at the time. (1997)

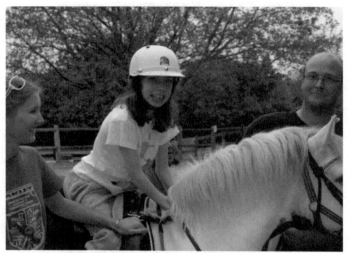

Horse riding at the South African Riding for the Disabled Association was one of my first loves. Volunteers always ensured I was safe and stayed in the saddle. (2005)

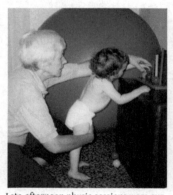

Late-afternoon physio sessions were our norm. This day was particularly warm and my physiotherapist, Eunice, wanted to see how my body was moving, so she stripped me down to my nappy. It was a win-win situation! (1996)

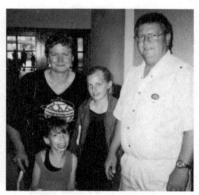

This is my family back in the day. (2003)

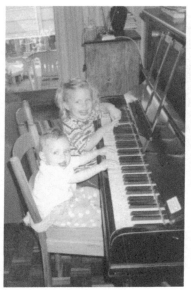

Sitting with Erin and playing the piano is a vivid memory for me. Good times. (1995)

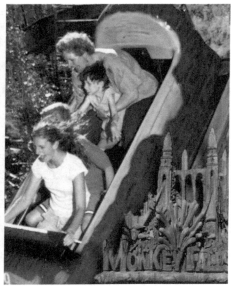

At Ratanga Junction riding my favourite thrill ride, Monkey Falls, with my mom and cousins during the school holidays. (2002)

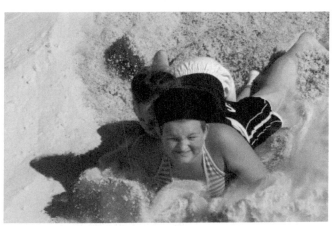

At Brownies I was included in everything, so when sandboarding was the activity of the day we found a way to make it happen for me too. My friend Lisa and I had a blast that day! (2005)

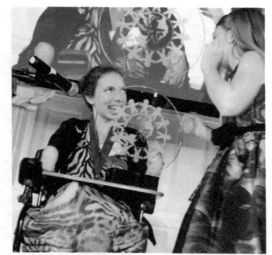

Receiving the World of Children Youth Award in New York. (2013)

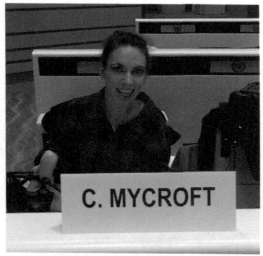

My first time speaking at the United Nations in Geneva. This made my activist heart so happy. (2016)

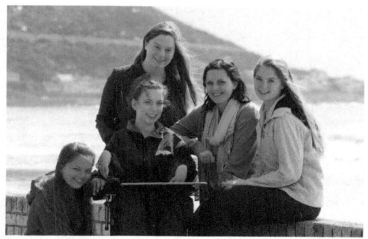

The founders of The Chaeli Campaign: Chelsea, me, Tarryn, Erin and Justine.
I'm so grateful for these powerhouse women. (2011) (Photo: Roy Beusker)

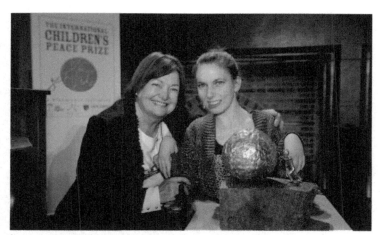

The awesome Mairead Maguire was the Nobel Peace Laureate who handed over
my International Children's Peace Prize. (2011) (Photo: KidsRights Foundation)

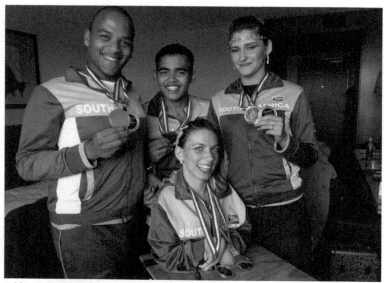

Celebrating with Damian, Mukkie and Chantelle after becoming double world champions at the Holland Dans Spektakel. (2015)

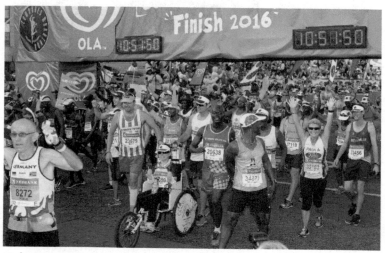

My first time crossing the Comrades Marathon finishing line. Hudson, Lepel and I finished in a time of 10 hours and 51 minutes. (2016)

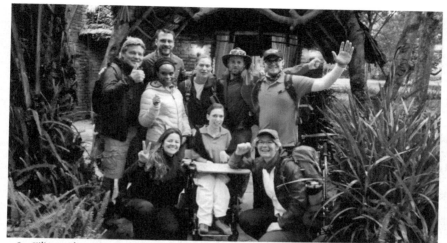

Our Kili team the morning we started climbing the mountain. Back: Danie, Thembi, Adam, Sally, Carel and Taylor. Front: Johanna, me and Anne. (2015)

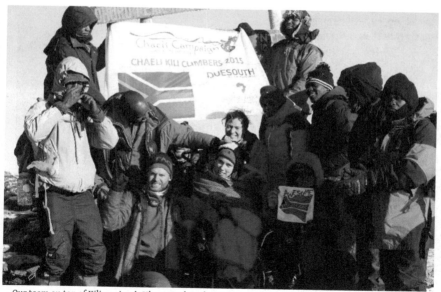

Our team on top of Kilimanjaro's Uhuru Peak with our Summit Africa guides. We were freezing, but so excited that we had made it. (2015)

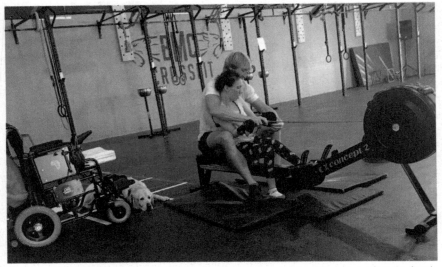

My first time figuring out how to use my legs on the rowing machine in a CrossFit session with Marco. (2018)

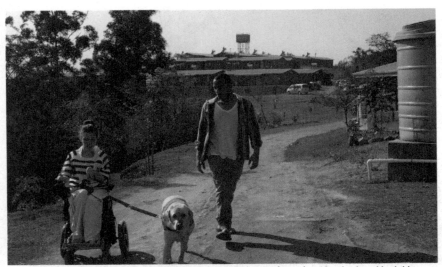

We did inclusion workshops with LIV Village in Durban, which cares for orphaned and vulnerable children. Here I am exploring with Damian and Eden. (2015)

PART 2: ACTIVE AND ABLE ADVENTURES

Chapter 5
The makings of an adventurer

It has been such an incredible journey figuring out how to navigate life with my disability and living it to the full. It has certainly not always been easy and some lessons have been hard to learn. Some of them I'm still learning, which is half the journey, right? We've always approached my life like this: if we decide to do something but we're not 100% sure how to make it happen or how it's going to go, that's okay. We'll figure it out as we go and we just need to trust that it's going to work out for the best.

The Chaeli Campaign has been an adventure in itself. It has led us down a path that has introduced us to some remarkable people who are so passionate about what they do and are making a positive impact in the communities they serve. I can't imagine my life without these wonderful people. I am so proud and grateful that our work has created opportunities for me to do some of the most rad things I've ever experienced with people who live out the ethos and message of The Chaeli Campaign in the best possible ways.

It's crazy to think about how my life has changed through becoming more active (the mainstream understanding of the word). I have had to grow in so many ways, most of which have very little to do with my body and physical wellbeing. It's been a journey of finding new parts of myself – parts I didn't know I had – and doing things I didn't know I was capable of doing. Maybe that's a small untruth, as I've always felt that I'm capable, I just didn't always allow myself to explore all the opportunities to get involved so that I could put that capability to the test, probably because I was scared. I get annoyed with myself that I was afraid, because look at what happened – I have had some of the most exciting, liberating (and terrifying) life experiences since I embraced that fear. Now, don't get me wrong, I'm not always a fearless person, ready to take on every adventure anyone suggests. It's a process, a work in progress...

I can't see it as a problem because not being able to do things alone means that I now have so many shared experiences – experiences that have had a profound impact on those who have shared them with me. I mean, if you ask any of my partners about our adventures, there is one constant, namely crying. You'll see...

I'M AN INVESTOR

I have the most incredible people accompanying me on this journey, uncovering my inner adventurer. Putting all these lessons down on paper and thinking about these ridiculous, unbelievable humans who have found their way into my life in beautiful ways (sometimes with the craziest coincidences – if you believe in coincidences), understanding these lessons at a deeper level and realising the impact they've had on me is quite a task. We don't always know we're having a profound experience while it's happening. It's only when I give myself an opportunity to reflect on them, such as now when I am sharing these stories with you, that the magnitude of it all sinks in.

Building strong relationships is fundamental to me being able to do all the things I do. It's a crucial skill I've had to learn to embrace my potential. It has taken me a long time to be okay with having a small group of friends and supporters. You don't need hundreds or thousands of people to make things possible, you just need a few really good ones. I learnt this on our journey with The Chaeli Campaign and I keep learning it every time I take on new challenges and adventures. In reaching this point of acceptance I have also recognised that I'm an investor. I invest so much of myself in building these strong relationships that I've got very deep connections with each of the people in my support circle. I hold them close and cherish them.

Sometimes I feel like I'm too much for people, and I need to be reminded that if they didn't want to be around, they wouldn't be. And I think this deep investment mentality comes from a feeling of wanting and hoping and believing in that same level of investment from others. It has a lot to do with my disability and how much energy it consumes – I need to remember that these bags are heavy and they get easier to carry when I share the load. See, what gets to my overthinking brain (thoughts I'm constantly working on shutting down) is the thought that my disability makes it harder to connect, and people don't want to work that hard. I counter this thought with a question to myself. What if my disability is the avenue to true connection with others? What if I show up, wholeheartedly, in all my disabled glory...? What adventures could that lead to?

Let's take a second to breathe before all of the ridiculousness of living my life, active and able. As I started unpacking these memories and stories I realised that every step and turn has led to a new challenge and new points of growth, learning and expanding what it means to live fully, focusing on my ability and sharing it with those around me. So I figure the best way to approach this part of my story is to discuss the era in terms of the "active and able" partners I have had, and the special lessons I've learnt from – and with – them, while having some of the most epic moments in my life.

Before I dive into these relationships and their impact on me, I want to share some fundamentals to keep in mind as we go through these stories.

FUNDAMENTALS OF ADVENTURE

"Adventure" is often sold to us as something that only some people can do, or something that requires a certain body type or personality. I don't agree. Adventures are pretty much always a challenge in some way. So if an adventure is aligned with taking on a challenge, and I face challenges on the daily, then every day can be seen as an adventure!

It is easier and more entertaining for me to see my everyday challenges as an adventure rather than seeing my days as being filled with challenges. This is not to say that every day I'm a motivation station brimming with positivity. What makes the idea of an adventure exciting is often the challenge itself and not always how difficult an activity is. There are so many instances where we're making amazing (and often hilarious) memories and learning life lessons along the way.

I believe that adventurers are born *and* raised.

Some people are always looking for new and exciting epic things to do. Others have to learn how to take a leap outside their comfort zone. I think my disability gives me a good balance between the two. There are things that are definitely more of a struggle, requiring more logistical, practical support because I'm disabled – even so-called "normal" activities. I'm so grateful that I've always been encouraged to do the "normal" things that non-disabled people do with minimal, if any, planning or strategising.

Things that are often seen as mundane and simple, like playing the piano with my sister when I was a toddler, became adventures because we had to make a plan to make it happen. I was tiny and had no balance. I could barely reach the keys, but I wanted to play the piano. We used a long scarf tied around me and the back of the chair to make sure I was relatively safe, and there we were, making music and memories.

The push to get involved in advocacy and awareness-raising has often been after arriving somewhere to do something fun and then discovering it wasn't accessible or finding that the people in charge didn't want me to take part because I was in a wheelchair. Advocacy comes in many different shapes and sizes, and most times in my life it has taken the form of action. My family and friends have made things possible by *doing* them. Most of the time, people are fearful of things going wrong, so they just say no. We have always combated this fear by doing the things; showing that these fears are based on flawed ideas.

Just like when I spoke about my experiences at high school and about people having different understandings and interpretations of what is reasonable, "possibility" faces similar challenges. The big problem here is that, more often than not, the people deciding on policies – policies are a huge barrier – have a relatively narrow view of what is or what should be possible because disabled people aren't included in the discussions as we should be. It's easier to just say that disabled people can't do something (read: not allowed to do something) than it is to find a creative solution to ensure we can participate and be included. This is also impacted by the fact that people don't want to be held liable if something goes wrong.

My family, friends and I have never bought into the idea that I couldn't do stuff. Obviously there are certain practical things that I physically can't do, but that doesn't make experiences entirely unattainable or unachievable. This has always made our stories more entertaining because when you add disability logistics to any situation, it's bound to become more interesting and complicated.

I'm so happy I've had the opportunity to do some rad, random things. I've been on top of fire engines, ridden camels, fallen off ostriches (in hindsight, this one may have been a slight error of judgement), donkeys and horses. I've done bumper cars with Justine sitting with me in the same car – we had to do some convincing here, but we got it right. I have also done the spinning teacup thing. I sat on my uncle's lap for this and I was so nauseous on that ride that I was crying within 30 seconds of it starting. It lasted the longest four minutes of my life and after throwing up I decided I never needed to do that again. It's not a disabled thing, it's just a me thing.

When I was younger, we went to Ratanga Junction – a theme park in Cape Town – a few times, and we'd go on some of the thrill rides. It's closed down now, but we had some great times there. Monkey Falls, a waterfall ride with a fall of 18,5m and one of the highest waterfall rides in the world, was by far my favourite ride. Once, we waited in line for ages and as we reached the front the people who worked there were a bit perplexed about the wheelchair and how it would fit into the "log". After we explained that the wheelchair didn't need to come with us, they were much more accommodating. So much so that when we came back around after the ride was done, they asked us if we wanted to go again instead of getting out and standing in line again. Um, yes, thank you! We did that ride eight times in a row that day and it was awesome. I think I was about eight years old and I still remember it vividly.

We didn't go to this theme park very often and after such a great, inclusive experience, we figured it would be that way every time. Not so much. When we went back a year or so later the park had changed its policies and no longer allowed people with physical or mental disabilities to go on any of the thrill rides.

I have been raised with a propensity for adventure, and we would always embrace the moments where we could do something fun, even when policies are exclusionary and discriminatory. When we found out about this particular policy change, we requested to sign a waiver or something, but no such document was available and there was no alternative solution. It turned out that this was the policy in theme parks across South Africa, which is a pity considering that we had already proven that it is possible to use these rides safely as a disabled person.

Fast-forward a number of years and we were in Los Angeles for work for Chaeli Foundation USA (this was the same trip where we had the airport bathroom debacle) and had a free day, so we went to Universal Studios, and had a completely different experience. When we arrived I was fully expecting not to be allowed to do anything that was vaguely exciting. I was wrong. Universal Studios has a system where you decide which experiences you'd like to do, and you then get time slots so that they know where and when you're going to require assistance, and they make it happen. I was super excited about this, and just being accommodated in that way was cool. We did the studio tour and I was strapped in safely, in my wheelchair, with no issues. I've been on low-key thrill rides, but never a ride that would classify as a roller-coaster. My size usually disqualifies me and, I must say, I had never really had a problem with not being able to go on the fast-moving, topsy-turvy, scream-inducing rides. I was fine with staying safely in my wheelchair for those.

But when we were inside Harry Potter World and someone suggested we go on the ride there, reassuring us that there was a disability-friendly version that was still a good time, I was keen to give it a go. This was quite possibly the most terrifying moment of my mother's life...

So we went through a darkened passage that felt like we were heading to a dungeon-type place. I was nervous and excited. They asked me if I was able to sit upright on my own and I responded with a yes – and the only other information we received about this ride was that we were going to be using the "stationary seats". The ride operator put his hand against the wall and, magically, a set of seats arrived for us to get into. We were trusting this ride and these people with, frankly, very little information and it was arguably pretty reckless. Anyway, Mom took me out of my wheelchair and put me in the telephone-booth-shaped seat compartment vibe and left the wheelchair with the operator. This booth had a big pommel that went between your knees and the usual pull-down safety thing, so I felt I was securely in there. At the last minute Mom kicked off her shoes and they landed next to my wheelchair. Smart move.

I think I have a *vastly* different interpretation of the word "stationary". See, to me, if you refer to something as being stationary, I understand that to mean that whatever that thing is, it does not or will not move. I realised this difference in understanding about five seconds into the ride when, all of a sudden, we were upside down and spinning around, chasing Harry Potter on a broomstick! It was the most intense ride I've ever been on in my life. The first time we went upside down, my ass left the seat and I freaked out (without making a sound). I was in shock. A second later I had to have a conversation with myself to remind myself that I did actually have some control over my body.

The thing is, once you're on it there's no turning back or stopping. You have to be there for the duration of the ride. So we were on this ride... I couldn't see Mom and she couldn't see me (because of the phone booth set-up), apart from my flailing little legs when we went around corners. I was processing the fact that I was being flung around at great speed, upside down, and had no other option but to hang in there, so I was focused on keeping myself grounded, pressing my bum into my seat and bracing myself for the movements (it was quite the workout), and Mom was contemplating how she was going to explain to our family that I had died, having fallen out of the seat on a Harry Potter ride. I had the *best* time! When we rolled back into the station and they lifted the safety thing, Mom came around to me fully expecting to find me a complete mess of panicked tears – based on my spinning teacup encounter – but I was laughing hysterically. I think she was kind of annoyed that I had been having the time of my life while she had been stressing her heart out.

Mom put me back in my chair. I was beaming (I totally think I was overstimulated, though) and she was exhausted. That was the last thing we did at Universal Studios. We went back to our hotel, where Mom said she needed a nap after that experience. She's also told me since that she has no issues with me going on rides like that, but I need to find somebody else to go with me because her mom heart can't take it. I'm okay with that. New adventure buddies!

HORSE POWER

I've always loved animals. I was obsessed with watching all the shows on Animal Planet and for a long time I wanted to be a zoologist. So, when I had the opportunity to go to the South African Riding for the Disabled Association (SARDA) and be able to interact with these animals on a regular basis, I was so happy. Obviously, there are also all of the physical, therapeutic benefits, but that wasn't a part of my reasoning. I was a part of their programme for six years and that's where I learnt that horses are remarkable, special beings. They have an ability to connect and understand in unique ways that make for beautiful relationships between horses and people.

I was six years old when I started riding and I loved it. When I started, I rode a horse named Flea (a petite female) but after a while my main horse was an old male named Chico. He was the best, the best gentleman of a horse. He was a retired police horse with a curved back and a beautiful soul. His back issue meant that he could only work with people who didn't weigh a lot, so we suited each other.

One day when I was getting onto Chico, the clipboard that was on the mounting ramp blew into his face. He freaked out, reared and stepped back away from the ramp before I'd had a chance to get a good grip on the reins and we'd put my feet in the stirrups. Chico quickly realised the situation and came back to centre and calmly continued through the lesson. He was always so aware and conscious of being careful. SARDA is a special place that does incredible work, with amazing volunteers and staff.

Chico's body eventually got too tired and his hind legs gave out, and he died a short time later. After that, riding wasn't the same for me. I rode other horses, but didn't feel as connected to what we were doing, even though I still loved it so much.

This all happened at the same time I was discovering wheelchair dancing. It became a bit of a struggle to balance both activities and there were time clashes, which made it even more difficult.
I had to make a decision as to whether I wanted to continue horse riding and only be able to go to half the dancing practices, or commit fully to the dancing and see where that new path would take me. I believe that

everything in life comes when it's needed. It's often unexpected, but it always leads to new adventures and lessons about yourself. I decided to commit to giving dancing more space in my life and I'm so glad I embraced it. It opened up a whole new world. (Cue the *Aladdin* soundtrack...)

In the same way that things happen as they must, life has taught me that things have a wonderful way of coming back around and bringing experiences full circle.

Most of my adventures I do to support the work of The Chaeli Campaign – raising funds through the activities and so on – and we were looking for something cool and crazy to raise funds and awareness, to change some perspectives and to challenge some stereotypes in the process of doing something rad and unexpected.

We worked with the King James Group, a world-class advertising agency, to make this next one happen. We discussed the objectives of a new, exciting adventure and challenge. They developed the concept "Bet Chaeli Can't", and came back to us with a list of epic ideas for me to choose from.

[TANGENT]
This is a good time to explain our relationship with King James so that this story makes more sense.

Mom has always been a total boss when it comes to networking and making connections. This time was no different. She met Alistair King, a founding partner of the agency, when I was two years old and she connected with him about King James potentially supporting the Western Cape Cerebral Palsy Association. At the time they were a fledgling company that only had three people working there and they just didn't have the capacity to do any pro bono jobs.

When we started The Chaeli Campaign seven years later, Mom remembered this connection (this is what makes her such a brilliant networker) and reached out again to see if there were any possibilities for partnership.

A meeting was organised to pitch our organisation to the agency directors to become one of their pro bono clients. Mom thought it a good idea for us, the five founders of The Chaeli Campaign, to deliver the pitch. Some may say this was a lot of pressure for five kids under the age of 12, but we revelled in it. I remember we felt very businesslike and did our presentation on a set of steps. (Looking back, this seems pretty symbolic, and steps also became an ongoing discussion between us, especially when a ramp was put in at their new premises. I'm told it's unofficially referred to as "Chaeli's ramp".)

We have been a pro bono client ever since, and are one of King James's oldest clients. Both directors, Alistair and co-founder James Barty, have been made Friends of The Chaeli Campaign – an honour we give to people who have gone above and beyond to support our work.

They've created the Chaeli Agency within the King James Group, which enables any employee to volunteer their time to work on our projects, and they can take on roles that are different from their everyday job titles. This is where "Bet Chaeli Can't" was born.
[TANGENT OVER]

The concept behind "Bet Chaeli Can't" was fundamentally about calling out the naysayers and encouraging people – if they didn't believe I could do the challenge – to put their money where their mouths were and to bet against me. They brought a whole bunch of ideas to the table, and we settled on a five-day endurance horse ride.

The challenge was to ride a horse for five hours a day for five days. Do you know how long that is when you're on a horse? I only realised fully on the first day. Oh my greatness, I was exhausted. And there were still four days to go.

We made a 45-second powerhouse promotional video and arriving at the studio to film was just epic. Everything was next-level and I felt more powerful simply just being in the space. That's when you know it's going to be good. We filmed for 14 hours, I think. I only cried once. (It's okay, the meltdown was a good stress release and I also feel that it made me more focused on what we were doing and getting it done.) If you think my eyes look a little red in one or two shots, that's why.

My focus for this was getting challenge-ready. I knew I would definitely have to put in work to have more stamina and strength for the whole endurance part. I figured that riding a horse would come back to me, like when you ride a bicycle. That didn't happen.

King James found a team of power women – Sarah, Jess, Georgia and Tash – to help make all the horse-related logistics happen, and I loved working with them.

The first thing to do was get me on a horse to see what would happen. I hadn't been on a horse in more than a decade and it showed. I forgot what a unique sitting position you have to have. Sisters Sarah and Jess had a majestic retired champion of a horse named Orpheus. We thought it would be smart to get a baseline to work with. Now, Orpheus had been retired for a good few years when I met him, and he was enjoying it. When I was helped onto his back (that was an adventure in itself, as he was a big, tall, broad boy) we all became slightly hysterical, as we discovered that I wasn't able to sit up the way you're supposed to on a horse because everything in my body that needed to be loose, wasn't. I hugged Orpheus properly that day.

We had our work cut out for us, but we were ready.

Sarah took the lead (see what I did there? Ha!) and found the best horse to partner us in this challenge. His name is Smokey and he lives at Mistico Equestrian Centre in the Cape Winelands. He was rescued with another horse. They discovered later that the other horse was pregnant and, when she had the foal, Smokey got quite attached to it even though it wasn't his. (Modern horse over here!) When the time came to decide how Smokey would spend the rest of his days, considering how he connected with the foals whenever they arrived, the team at Mistico decided that that would be his job. He is the stay-at-home dad and all the moms go out to work – dressage, jumping and so on – and this made me love him even more. I told you he's a modern horse. (There's no patriarchy at Mistico.)

I knew Smokey was a special horse. He gave me Chico vibes when it came to how intuitive and patient he was. From the moment I was on him, he knew I was a different kind of rider. We had a block we'd shaped to fit over the saddle so I could "rest" my arms on it and it was easier to sit up straight(er). We had devised an efficient plan to get me onto his back and were in the stalls, ready for my first proper ride. He wouldn't move.

It was almost as though he was saying, "Nope, this one isn't stable." (Ha, I did it again.) After some convincing he walked out of the stalls, so slowly that it barely registered as movement. As we had more sessions together he got more into it and learnt how we could work together. Every time we stepped off or onto a pavement, Smokey went slowly – one foot, a group check-in, verbal confirmation, and then the next foot; always considerate, making sure everyone was happy and comfy.

We trained together for months and during this time I started going to CrossFit, which helped immensely with my body being more comfortable while riding. When you choose to ride a horse, it's easy to forget that it's a living being and also has to be on board with the plan for it to be successful. You're a team. For this challenge, our team was just bigger, so we all had to be on the same page.

The five days officially started and we all learnt what a champion Smokey was. On the second day, we were walking around Joostenberg Vlakte outside Cape Town and walked past a house where, unbeknownst to us, a huge dog lived.

We were walking ahead of the King James crew, Mom was in the car and a couple of people were walking with us, filming everything. I was tied securely to the saddle, someone was walking on each side of me and someone was leading Smokey. We were laughing about something and it was all chilled until the dog jumped up against the gate. Smokey was spooked. He bolted forwards and across the road away from the gate. That felt like a smart move to me. However, in the process of panicking he had spun around and we found ourselves tangled up in some bushes. Within minutes Smokey realised, or remembered, that I, the unstable rider, was on his back and he calmed down. Those watching were worried, asking whether we were all okay. We were. I wasn't communicating with anyone. I think I was going over what had just happened and after replaying it once in my mind, I burst into anxious tears. I tend to have these reactions, often after the fact. People thought I was injured and went to get Mom.

"Chaeli's crying."

Mom, knowing our strategies, said, "It's okay, let's give her three minutes."

I realised I was fine – not injured, not dead, and still on the horse – and began some deep breaths so I could feel normal again and we could carry on. I don't know if that was caught on film, but if it was, I'd kind of like to see it.

After the adrenaline rush of the second day we were hoping for a relaxed day, but what would a Chaeli Challenge Adventure be without numerous moments of crisis?

Once again, we were so chilled, creating our own vibe. Then we heard a train in the distance. We were walking on a stretch of road that runs parallel to the train tracks and there were no side roads in sight. The train was coming. We didn't know how Smokey would respond but generally horses are not big fans of trains. We had to decide what to do. The consensus was to try to outrun the train. That sounds absurd to me as I write this. Who seriously thinks they can outrun a train? We did.

We thought there was enough distance between us and the train for us to at least get close to a side road, so that if Smokey did freak out when the train came past, we wouldn't have too much further to go. We were all on the same wavelength. My strategy for surviving this madness was just holding on for dear life.

When we started running, everyone around us was confused because that definitely hadn't been part of our training. We hadn't practised trying to outrun a train.

Those were some of the most intense minutes I've ever experienced. We thought Smokey would freak out, but he was the calmest of us all. He was just like, "Guys, why are we running? Ooh look, a train."

That was it. It clarified how unbelievable Smokey is. Sarah immediately phoned his owner, Siobhan, and when she answered, Sarah asked:

"Do you know how fucking phenomenal your horse is?!"

Siobhan, laughing, replied, "But of course!" And right then I knew we had underestimated so much about Smokey, based on what we understood to be the typical behaviour of horses. It felt like he was teaching us a life lesson...

Never underestimate someone or judge them based on how others have behaved in the past. Give them the benefit of the doubt.

By the last day, we were all obviously excited to be completing the challenge. We were also very much over trying to ride a horse for five hours a day for five days. Through the challenge we were raising funds for our Chaeli Cottage Inclusive Pre-School and Enrichment Centre and we were welcomed at the finish by all the children who attend the school. It was special to share that success with them.

The "Bet Chaeli Can't" campaign was a wonderful way of reconnecting with my love of horses. I hope that when reading this, you think back to something you've loved and left, and maybe find a way to rediscover it, all the while learning more about yourself.

I think it's about time to go and visit Smokey.

Dancing Away With My Heart

I was 11 years old when dancing became one of my main activities and sports. Admittedly, I did do ballet for about a second when I was little. Mom organised with Erin's ballet teacher to run classes that catered for me and a few other girls who also had CP. We did a lot of upper-body moves and routines where we were beautiful mermaids sitting on rocks. It was awesome that I could also don my tutu and do ballet. I have those memories too now, even though we didn't do it for that long.

One day we saw an article in the paper about Ballroom and Latin American wheelchair dancing, and we went to check it out. I was unsure about it and was totally okay with sitting on the side and watching, but the coach, Gladys Bullock, would have none of it. I remember her saying something like, "You didn't come here to sit, you came here to dance." After that lesson, I was hooked. Gladys is a true legend in inclusive dancesport in South Africa. She has been integral in bringing the sport to our country and I'm incredibly grateful to have had her lay the foundation of my dancing.

Ballroom and Latin American dancing suits my personality because I get to be classy and graceful for the Ballroom dances and I can also be sassy and spicy for the Latin American ones. (I think the graceful part is aspirational. I feel like I'm one of the clumsiest people around, but it's still a vibe.) With this sport, I get to express myself artistically while also embracing my competitive side. That works well for me.

I know many sports are done with teams and working closely with fellow athletes, but I think Ballroom and Latin American dancing are different in that the relationships built with partners are so personal. Partners are so important – you spend so much time together, building a strong connection and learning how each other works, that you share way more with them than any other person. I've had three dance partners in my dancing career.

Jesse
Jesse was my first official dance partner and we danced together for six years. He was three years older than me. We learnt a lot during that time. He was a really great partner to have when I was unsure of how to express myself as a dancer. Jesse has all the confidence, which allowed me to be shy and contained while I figured out the kind of dancer I

wanted to be. I appreciated that. Our partnership ended when I was in Grade 10 and this was a catalyst for us to start providing dance under the Chaeli Sports and Recreation Club (CSRC) – another of our non-profit organisations – and an opportunity to be part of growing inclusive dance in South Africa.

Brandon

Because of the years of work through The Chaeli Campaign, we had no issue finding disabled dancers. It's a difficult job to find standing partners who stay, and who are equally committed to building a dance partnership. This is an ongoing challenge for us, but it gives us the chance to be creative and find innovative solutions.

We decided that the best way of growing inclusive dance with the CSRC was to collaborate with dance schools that focused on non-disabled dance. We went to one of the well-known dance schools, Delta Dance Academy, and did a demo to show what wheelchair dancing is all about. Three amazing dancers joined us – Chantelle, Brandon and Damian. Chantelle now assists me in supporting our CSRC dancers and we share the responsibility for helping each dancer to fulfil their potential and reach their dancing goals.

After six months of not having a partner, I started dancing with Brandon. We were partners for just a season. Brandon did Ballroom but not Latin American, so I just did Ballroom for that year. I learnt during that time that I actually really love the Latin American dances and I wanted to do them again. We sat down and had a conversation about it and realised that we wanted different things. So, in a totally amicable way, our partnership ended with the season. I was sad about it because we had a good time as partners. It was an important moment for me, checking in with myself and recognising that it's okay to want different things and to go in new directions. We are still friends and see each other fairly often. Our friendship has survived the end of our dancing partnership and that's special.

Damian

My partnership with Damian just came to be, as though the universe knew we would make sense together as a dance couple. As my partnership with Brandon had come to an end, so had Damian's with his partner, Maggie, and there we were. I didn't quite understand how profound this relationship would be in my life and just how grateful I am to have had the privilege of knowing him.

We were dance partners for almost a decade, and spent hours and hours practising routines (and many hours doing nothing in particular). All of these hours that I thought I wasn't really paying attention to, or taking note of, have become so clear to me and I'm cherishing every minute.

The year 2020 was a year like no other. Nobody can disagree. As I write this we're still living through a global pandemic that has changed our lives, literally overnight. It ended with a blow I definitely wasn't ready for. Because of the lockdown regulations, we hadn't had dancing practice since March, but we'd restarted with a few of our CSRC dancers, obviously observing all the safety protocols. It felt like we were finding a way back to a semblance of normality and that we were going to be okay. The Covid-19 case numbers had begun increasing again and we had decided to finish our dancing year early, in November. Damian ran that last practice on his own because I was sick and woman down at home.

A couple of weeks later we received a message that Damian had been in a car accident and was in a coma. I read the message and instantly went pale and felt sick. I think that's happening again as I write this.

I never thought that I would be writing this story. I never imagined that there would be a time when he wouldn't be in my stories. I thought we would be together in our eighties, reminiscing about the good times. I guess that the story is meant to be different from what I've imagined.

I went into the mode of looking for the positives. He was on a ventilator. That wasn't necessarily a bad thing, I thought. It wasn't a great thing, but it was definitely not the worst. We didn't have a lot of information and people were asking me things because I was his partner, but there wasn't much I could share. We didn't know his status for a while. The next day we had some news – not great news, but you work with what you get – and as soon as we had heard about his injuries, I felt a little bit better because we could do something with that. I could let all of the people who had contacted me, asking what was going on, know what was going on. Because of Covid-19, we weren't able (or allowed) to go and see him, or to be there to support him or his family. So we had to do what we could from afar, which is not how we usually work in a crisis (not including the crisis of the pandemic, which is about staying home and staying safe).

There was so much communication within our club about sending prayers and positive, healing thoughts and energy to Damian and it really brought into focus that what we've built in our dancing club is a family. And one of our family members was struggling.

The first thing we found out was that the accident caused a brain injury and subsequent strokes. That was a lot to process, but I still believed Damian would be okay. Doctors were saying he was young and strong, which is a positive, right? After a week of ups and downs we understood that this was going to be a long journey. A couple of days after his accident, I said to Mom, "Whatever state he was in, it's fine. We can figure it out because he's still here."

I was ready to be that person who knows all the people working with him in his rehab, who always shows up to be supportive and bring the motivation. It wasn't like I hadn't waited for him to heal before...

[TANGENT]
Damian and I had been partners for just a few months. He was studying hospitality, something happened, and he fell and slipped a disc in his back. We couldn't dance for nine months while his back figured itself out. People asked me why I didn't look for a new partner and I was affronted. He was my partner and he was injured. It would be totally hypocritical for me to say goodbye because a part of his body currently wasn't working properly. And after nine months of waiting and rehab and work on his part, we were back on the dance floor.

I think this time was unbelievably good for us. It allowed us to get to know each other on a much deeper level, without the usual pressure of choreography and competition that is there when you're actually dancing. When we got back on the floor together we were so connected, it was as though we could read each other's minds.
[TANGENT OVER]

I don't think I have ever lived through a week that felt longer than that week after Damian's accident. Little did I know that the hours in a day were about to become excruciatingly long.

We were told that things had improved slightly (so we were feeling cautiously optimistic), but those improvements had turned into declines, and the following Saturday we found out that there was nothing more the doctors could do for him, and at about 10.30pm, Damian passed away.

I was watching a series when I got the message. Everyone in the house was sleeping. I called Mom and she came into my room. I asked her if she had seen the message and she hadn't, so I told her, but she either didn't hear or understand what I said. "He died!" I shouted. I've heard somewhere that it's important to say the words out loud, but I still didn't process what was happening. For 15 minutes or so I didn't do or say anything. I just stared at the paused series on my laptop screen, thinking it wasn't really happening. This wasn't the plan.

I wasn't prepared for this outcome, at least not at a conscious level. (The thought that he may not make it through this had passed through my subconscious, but my brain had stopped it from being too front-of-mind until it was absolutely necessary.) In some way, I'm grateful that he survived and fought for that week because it meant our grief could happen in almost manageable doses. I was thinking of all of the alternatives and the plans we would have to change as he recovered and the different ways we'd need to function to accommodate his new needs. If he wasn't able to communicate in the way we were used to, chilled. We already communicated largely without words anyway, so I wasn't too concerned about that. We could make a plan. But then he died. And all of those alternatives we were all devising became moot.

We were now thrust into making plans that didn't include him. I didn't want to be a part of these plans because that meant admitting he wasn't here. That was too much for me, especially for those first few weeks. I think one of the hardest things is changing how we speak about him – it's past tense now.

I always thought that if something tragic like this happened, I would be like a detective – looking for clues and answers to the millions of questions, and getting to the bottom of what happened. That hasn't been the case at all. I think I've been so shaken that any questions that were in my mind have been pushed aside because I subconsciously registered that spending all of my energy on questions wouldn't change anything. Knowing what happened that morning and having every detail of the accident won't bring him back to us. Sometimes having answers to questions doesn't bring closure or peace; sometimes answers just bring more questions.

About halfway through Damian's memorial, while I was listening to the tributes from his family, I was trying to focus on remembering to breathe and I had some intrusive thoughts that I tried desperately, and unsuccessfully, to block out.

"I don't want to be here. This is so hard."

I was asked to speak at the memorial, but I couldn't even think about Damian without bursting into tears, so Mom spoke on behalf of our dance family. She decided to end with the tribute I'd posted to my social media. It showed everyone the Damian that we knew and loved. I was broken listening to those words that were so difficult to write, but it was perfect.

[MY TRIBUTE TO DAMIAN]
I don't know how to sum up our partnership, or what it's meant in our lives. It's been profound. I'm not going to say it's over because I believe what we learnt together and from each other lives on, even though we're in different places now.

We had our own language that confused so many, but we didn't care; it didn't matter. We knew what we were doing and most of the time we didn't need words. You have been one of the best-hearted humans I've ever met and you lit up every room and space you entered and made an impact in every one of them.
The best were the small moments. Falling asleep on your shoulder on long flights; playing random music without any plan and "accidentally" devising a new dance move we loved. You embraced your whole self and you always encouraged me to embrace all my capabilities when I was unsure, promising you would never let me fall, and keeping your promise.

Dancing with you was my safe space and there are few places I've felt more empowered and fulfilled than with you by my side on a dance floor. I'm grateful to have shared so many years with you in my life, partner.

We've lost an impeccable, irreplaceable person.

"I'm sorry for your loss..." These words are designed to bring comfort and show compassion. The outpouring of love and support we have received from all around the world has been remarkable and it's truly appreciated. It also makes it harder, though, because every time I hear those words or a variation of them it reminds me of the loss we've experienced, and continue to experience. I know that people say that time heals all wounds, but I don't think enough time has passed for me to not feel like I've been hit in the face.

My body can take a second to receive or listen to a message that my brain is sending. I've realised that this doesn't only happen to me when I'm trying to do something active with my body; it is also when I am processing life and how I'm processing this loss. My mind remembers that he's not here any more, but my heart forgets, and then belatedly remembers. Suddenly I can't breathe.

I lost a best friend that day. I always thought people were being dramatic when they said they were heartbroken. I always thought it was a metaphor. I now know this kind of loss is indeed a physical experience.

I miss everything about Damian. His uncontrollable laughter still rings in my head. I hear a song or see a video that has something I think would be cool to add to a dance and I reach for my phone to send it to him. I forget for a split second.

In the days following Damian's death, I tried not to think about it. This was a terrible idea. I was non-functional. After the memorial I realised why that wasn't working. He is everywhere. Everywhere I look in our home there is a picture, a medal, a trophy, an accidentally kept hotel-room key from one of our trips. It's impossible to escape from him. I've realised that this is not a bad thing. It's such a blessing that we had him in our lives for the time we did, and the fact that we have constant reminders of his value and presence in our lives is just that – a reminder. And I've had to reset my mind to take in these reminders. Instead of focusing on how overwhelmingly sad I am that people who join my life story from here on out won't get to meet him, that we won't be making any more memories, I can cherish those moments when we created them. He was a gift and had an uncanny ability to make everyone around him smile. When we watch videos of him now, especially of him dancing, and when we tell stories about him, we can't help but smile. That was like his superpower. His presence would always lift the mood and spirit wherever he was. This was a beautiful thing because he worked so hard to find that happiness for himself, and all that work led to him being a beacon of joy for the rest of us.

So, this is what I'm choosing to take forward: the joy Damian brought all of us and how much he impacted people's lives – so much more than he ever knew (or admitted). I hope he knows now.

He was a compass I didn't know I had. Not in a guiding way, but more in a grounding way. Whatever was going on in my life, he was a constant, an unconditional constant. Now that he's not here, there is an unfillable space that we have to figure out how to navigate life with.

My last real conversation with Damian (not including the usual banter) was so typical of our relationship. I hadn't seen him in seven months because of the pandemic and the lockdown and social-distancing protocols. The hall was buzzing and we all felt weirdly normal. I was sitting on my own before we started the class. Damian walked in with his usual nonchalance. We made eye contact and he walked over to me with more enthusiasm than he normally would. We hugged for about a minute. It was a proper hug.

Some seconds of silence went by and I said, "I missed you."

He replied, "I missed you too."
He gave his trademark chuckle but didn't let go. After another 15 seconds or so of silent hugging, Damian said, "We're doing a demo. Let's go dance."

A few new people were joining us for the first time and we always did demos to show what we do, and what's possible. We hadn't danced together for those seven months and I was nervous that I wouldn't remember any of our routines. The thing is, when you have a partnership like ours, the second I looked at him I knew what we were doing. Even if it wasn't exactly the routine we had practised all those months before, we made it look like it was. The last dance we did was a rumba, the dance of love. And looking at how everything has turned out, I feel like that was a fitting last dance.

We had so many good times, great memories, and I'll share a few from our international dance moments.

We fought like an old married couple. When you spend so much time together, you're bound to get on each other's nerves. We also laughed constantly. I think that's what we did most, and I love that. I think we were able to laugh so much because we really understood each other in a special way. I believe that we all have many soulmates – people who are meant to be in our life – and I think he was one of mine.

Much of our time during practices (in between perfecting routines and choreography, of course) was spent talking about our lives, our plans for the future and our thoughts and feelings about all kinds of things. Damian was always ready to listen and give space for my venting, and to offer insights that I hadn't considered. I did the same for him. I think what made our partnership so special was that we both knew the other had baggage and things they were working through, and in acknowledging this we gave each other the freedom to be exactly who we were, in all our flawed, messy, beautiful glory.

When we started dancing together I was dancing Ballroom in a standard dancing wheelchair and Latin American in my motorised wheelchair. This isn't really how people do it, but hey, life is a journey. It took a few years to build my confidence and find the beauty and skill in fully committing to dance everything in the motorised chair. Thinking back, I'm not sure why I was so hesitant about switching to doing it all in the motorised chair. Maybe a part of me felt as though it would be "admitting" that my ability level wasn't as high as I thought it was. I have since recognised that going all in on this actually gives me more ability to show my skill, not less. I can also use my motorised wheelchair in unique ways to show people that they shouldn't underestimate my ability and my strength. Damian played a massive part in my accepting this and embracing it wholeheartedly.

We competed overseas a few times, at the Holland Dans Spektakel. I had been once before in 2008 with Jesse, and going back was an amazing experience. It was like a family reunion. And every time we went back, it had that feeling. Yes, we were there to compete and when we were at the competition venue that was the focus, but at the hotel, in the bus on the way to the venue or to and from the airport, it was all love and one of the most supportive dance experiences I've had. We built very special international friendships.

The first time I competed on the world stage with Damian was in 2014. What a learning curve! We received the programme for the competition and saw that there were 17 couples in our section alone, and we were shocked. In South Africa, we don't have that level of competition in terms of numbers. (We're working on this.) So, when our section wasn't a straight final (with the top six couples) and instead started with rounds, we knew we had to fight for a place on the podium. It was so exciting and so terrifying all at the same time. We placed second in Latin American and seventh in Ballroom that year. We caused quite a stir because we did things with the motorised wheelchair that nobody there had seen before and that were deemed impossible – until we hit the floor and proved them wrong.

Damian was incomprehensibly strong, in more ways than one. He was able to do things like lift my wheelchair with such ease and grace, which quite honestly regularly left me flabbergasted. His big, broad chest (and the way he carried himself on the dance floor) made him intimidating to many of our competitors... They didn't realise that it was just making room for his big heart.

I trusted him with my entire being. This was obviously important in our dancing, but I think it translated into our dancing routines too because I trusted him with my whole self – my heart and soul too – off the floor as well. He never let me fall. He would put his own body on the line to make sure that I always felt safe and brave. You can achieve many incredible things when you feel that sense of security.

The last local competition we did before the 2014 Holland Dans Spektakel was a complete disaster. Everything leading up to us getting onto the floor was normal, but then we got on the floor and things started to fall apart... The waltz was solid. It was the only thing that was solid in that day's dance performance. There was added pressure because before we started dancing, it was announced that we were going to represent South Africa in the Netherlands. During the tango, we discovered on our first fast turn that the balance of my chair was not quite centred and I tipped over backwards. This is generally not that big of an issue because we can just counterbalance and everything's fine. This time, though, I'd gone too far over and in trying to get back to centre, I fell diagonally and it was much more problematic to fix. The music then changed to a Viennese waltz and it was pretty much business as usual. Nothing dramatic happened. We moved on to the slow foxtrot, under the impression that our luck had changed, when midway through this dance my safety wheel (the little wheel that sits in the middle to stabilise the chair) decided it no longer wanted to serve its purpose and fell off in the middle of the dance floor. At this point I had almost reached breaking point, but we still had the quickstep to go, to finish off the section. I had basically no trust in my wheelchair and we were about to do the fastest dance, the dance that requires the most energy and the happiest face. How do you think it went?

Not well, people! It was like a comedy of errors. A very small part of me found it funny. Every time a new thing went wrong, it became increasingly less funny. Every time I looked at Damian he was sending me messages like, "It's fine, just keep going." We truly embodied the mantra "the show must go on" that day. We had to keep it together for the amount of time we were on the floor. That's about eight minutes. It felt like eight hours to me. When we got off the floor Damian knew I was just about to crack and completely lose it. As soon as someone said "Well done!" to us, I burst into tears. He hugged me as I cried and smudged my makeup all over his white shirt. It's moments like this that bring us together. So they say. We discovered once I had gathered myself and the adrenaline had run out that in the chaos I had sprained my elbow.

We left for the Netherlands four days later. It probably wasn't the best decision for my elbow, to compete at international level with an injury like that, but I embraced the "show must go on" mantra, and we did pretty well. I rested my arm when we got home for a good few weeks to take care of it.

I remember one of our competitors, Tim from the Netherlands, told me after the competition, "We can all see how much respect he has for you." I hadn't thought about it specifically until that moment, but our partnership was always rooted in mutual respect and I believe that's what made us strong. Many of the dancers and their supporters would watch us while we were dancing. One dancer was chatting to Mom during dinner and Damian started feeding me because we knew Mom was invested in the conversation. When we got up to get some dessert, the dancer told Mom that my partner was amazing. He said, "Damian shows people how to be a partner, just by being her partner." When I think about that now, I appreciate how simple yet profound and true that statement was.

He has changed so many minds just by being who he was, and to me that shows how truly powerful he was.

We became double world champions in our section the following year, in 2015. That was possibly one of the moments I have felt most fulfilled on the dance floor. Everything fell into place for us to make it happen, and it was glorious. We shared this moment with our friends and fellow dancers, Chantelle and Mukhtar (we call him Mukkie), who also became double champions in their section. South Africa showed up that year and we had a 100% success rate. We had the best adventures that year.

We had planned to go back to defend our title in 2016. Actually, because Damian and I and Chantelle and Mukhtar had both won the Latin American and Ballroom sections in our respective classes/categories based on disabilities, we would be promoted to the next level, World Cup, the next time we competed internationally. We were excited about this opportunity to up our game. When it came time to enter, we did just that, but a few months before the competition we realised we hadn't saved or raised enough funds for the whole team, to cover the cost of travelling to the Netherlands as well as our accommodation.

The KidsRights Foundation, the international children's aid and advocacy organisation based in Amsterdam in the Netherlands that awards the International Children's Peace Prize, connected with us to find out whether we would have any time available to do some talks and dance demos before the competition, and we told them that sadly we were no longer able to take part in the competition. They agreed to cover the shortfall for me, Damian and Mom so that we could travel to the Netherlands. We would arrive a few days earlier to support some of their initiatives. It was an amazing trip. It turned out to be our last overseas trip with Damian, and I'll cherish that forever.

That trip was one of many lessons, both taught and learnt. Damian and I wanted to explore the city a little while Mom stayed at the hotel. We had no idea where we were going, so we just walked everywhere. We got hopelessly lost looking for an Albert Heijn supermarket, and some lovely people assisted us with directions to the nearest one.

Getting back with all our shopping bags was an adventure too. We had a couple of the bags on the back of my wheelchair and Damian was holding a couple too. We left the supermarket and as we walked past another shop, we heard them playing a song that sounded like a paso doble. We were all alone in this beautiful square and we decided, "Why not?" So Damian put the bags down and we danced a paso doble, right there. We weren't paying attention to anything other than each other and doing that paso with all of our energy, and when we looked up there was a group of four or five people who had gathered to watch us and find out what we were doing. That's what makes dance beautiful. Dance can happen wherever the inspiration strikes, and when you're with people who have the same understanding. It was such a random and cool thing to have happened. It felt as though we were in a dance movie for a quick second, and that felt awesome. The most memorable moments are sometimes the moments that come without a warning.

Many of the people were confused by our relationship and how we communicated with each other. Often our communication was non-verbal and when it wasn't we were blatantly honest with each other, especially when we were irritating each other. At the competition that year our communication strategy was quite obvious and resulted in many curious eyes and questions. We were so secure in our partnership by this stage that anybody questioning our stability as a couple was a great distraction from the nerves we were both feeling.

This time there was pressure because we had been so successful the previous year, plus it was our first time in the professional section. We also found out when we arrived at the venue that our photo was on the entrance tickets...

Let me paint a picture for you.

Damian and I had completely different ways of preparing and getting into the right mental space for competition. He always wanted to warm up and run through routines with full focus and energy, but I don't work that way. I like to keep things light and chilled, and to run through routines just to feel the floor. It's the only space in my life when I don't try to overthink what I'm doing. What this meant for our partnership was that we couldn't prepare together. We sat a few seats apart and did our own thing, and when we came together on the floor, we were ready to dominate.

For this particular competition we were doing none of the above. I don't know why. So we were warming up on the floor and Damian was more nervous than usual, and when he was nervous, his stress manifested in him becoming a little patronising and bossy. (We knew this from previous experiences, so we'd manage it.) I remember he said something like, "You're not being committed to this." Since we'd been awake since about 5am, that felt like a pretty unfair statement to me. I knew it was nerves talking because I was feeling them too, and in the calmest tone I could muster, I took a breath, looked up at him and said, "Partner, I'm walking away from you now." Then I left the floor like a diva. We didn't talk about that interaction for the rest of the competition day. We moved on; we had bigger things to focus on and we were totally fine, but I can see why some people might have been concerned about the status of our partnership. That evening, when we were chilling in our hotel room with a drink, we spoke through what had happened and cleared the air. Damian said, "But Chaels, when I get like that, you just need to tell me to calm the fuck down."

I took that info on board and the next day we put it to the test. It was a more stressful day because we didn't do as well as we had hoped in the Ballroom section. (We came seventh, which was still pretty stellar, but we were nevertheless disappointed.) We wanted to do better in the Latin American section, and because of this pressure Damian was starting to get sucked into the same stress spiral as the day before. Instead of leaving the floor I moved to a different spot and as I walked away from him, I said, "Damian, calm the fuck down." And he did. That was the strategy we always followed after this and eventually we didn't even have to use words. It was all in the eyes.

Memories like these have a special place in my heart and always will. They try to fill the space that Damian did. Memories like these can also be brutal. I know that I will move forward with them and it's going to get easier to talk and think about him without falling apart, but moving forward also means living through the moments that bring all of the memories flooding back. I'm getting ready for all of the firsts – the first time we go to a competition without him, the first time I hear a song that we loved dancing to, and so many more.

Every time we came back home after competing, we had grown as dancers and we learnt so much that we could bring back to our CSRC dancers. Our dance family is a diverse melting pot of people with all kinds of challenges and skills. We are magical and often ridiculous. We focus on having fun while being excellent.

Dancing is such an incredible opportunity to express yourself and to do things that you never thought possible. I've been a dancer longer than I haven't and it's not just something you do with your body, it lives in you and comes through your soul. Everyone should have something like this in their life that brings them joy.

Chapter 6
Making history with a whole lot of firsts

CAN I EVEN RIDE A BICYCLE?

My initial response to this question? Nope...

Going way back, I had a tricycle, and the mandatory toddler motorbike. I wasn't coordinated enough to move forwards on that motorbike, so I just reversed everywhere. Maybe that's part of the reason I'm good at parallel parking. When I was a little older I had a bigger tricycle, as we know balance has never been my best attribute, and we adjusted it so that it didn't go backwards whenever I spasmed. (I'm pretty sure there's an actual mechanical term for this.) But I always looked at my tricycle as part of therapy for my hip joints and so on, and it took forever for me to ride anywhere. I never really classified cycling into the "fun" or "recreational" category of activities; it was more in the "necessary evil" category for me. So, when Grant (I'll tell you more about him shortly) first asked me whether I wanted to cycle with him, I was sceptical.

Clearly it was a good experience because I've now done the Cape Town Cycle Tour a good number of times, and the 94.7 Cycle Challenge once. (I'm not so keen to do that one again!)

Grant (also known as "G")
My introduction to Grant needs an explanation and it also reveals why it is important to include all key stakeholders in all conversations concerning them, to avoid serious confusion.

I was in matric and we were writing prelims. I had just finished writing a History exam and was sitting outside school waiting for someone to fetch me. I often think this could have been an orchestrated situation because it seems too coincidental that the day I met him, whoever was supposed to be picking me up was horribly late. Nobody has confirmed or denied this.

185

Anyway, I was sitting there, annoyed that I had been forgotten, and some random dude on a bicycle, in full cycling gear, rode past, went around the circle and parked his bike next to me. I thought this was weird. Who was this person? I'm relatively used to random people coming up to me and starting a conversation because when you're disabled people do this often, for some reason. This was different because it felt purpose-driven, like he had ridden his bicycle there specifically to speak to me. I don't remember how the conversation started because I was confused by the whole situation. There was probably a judgy hello from my side and subsequent awkward interactions. I'm pretty sure he didn't introduce himself, and I didn't get too much other information. But I do remember that he said this: "I have a proposal for you, but I need to speak to your mom first."

This was met with a confused look from me, and he said I should have a good day further (or something to that effect) and that he would be in touch. Then he left on his bike.

What was even happening? What did he mean? (I've never met you, and now you arrive outside my school and in 15 seconds you have a "proposal"?)

Naturally, I wanted to speak to people about this encounter, but I didn't really know what to say. What did he look like? I didn't know – he looked like a cyclist. As it turned out, I had actually met him before, but again, he was in cycling gear and we probably only interacted for about 10 minutes. I'm now much better at recognising cyclists because I've learnt what to look for. Mostly, I recognise people by looking at their legs/calf muscles (I'm close to the ground in my buggy, so this is my frame of reference) – they're a little like a cyclist's fingerprint.

The next day, when Mom picked me up from school, she told me we were going to the little café at Steenberg Village to meet someone. I figured it was someone who wanted to work with us for a Chaeli Campaign project, but it was the random dude on the bicycle from the previous day. Mom and Grant were clearly in cahoots. (Grant's dad, Gary, had learnt about our work and had made a plan to introduce Grant to us with the idea of him collaborating with us.) I wasn't included in this plan-making stage, probably because I had said no to cycling before and I guess Mom wanted to give Grant a fighting chance. Good call, I reckon.

Grant's pitch was basically: "Why not ride the Cape Town Cycle Tour with me? I'm a solid cyclist. What's the worst that can happen?" In my mind, there's a lot that can happen; so many worst-case scenarios, all entirely possible. I don't know what convinced me to say yes. It wasn't his pitch because that clearly needed some work... Actually, that's not true. I know what convinced me. It was his face. He's pretty beautiful.

I later discovered that as clichéd as it may sound, he's as beautiful on the inside as he is on the outside. (He's probably blushing as he reads this.)

So I had committed to riding the Cape Town Cycle Tour with this person. We connected over our mutual love for Taylor Swift, so we knew what our cycling playlist was going to be. It was the one thing we didn't need to have a conversation about. We didn't know anything about each other and we had no plan for how we were going to execute the whole thing. We knew we had to find something that I could be pulled in because these legs of mine were not going to get me through 109km.

[TANGENT]
The day I had coffee with Grant and agreed to cycle with him was the same day I went back to my old high school for the first time since leaving. There was a cricket final and my uncle's team was playing, so we went to support them. I can't help but feel that this has some profound significance. It almost felt as though two eras in my life met, and one was put to bed so that I could move forwards with the new one.
[TANGENT OVER]

Luckily for us, I'm relatively good at researching stuff. I'm relentless and persistent when it comes to finding a solution. We started searching for what we decided was called "a buggy". All the other options felt too patronising. We knew it was possible because Team Hoyt (father Dick, who sadly passed away in March 2021, and his son Rick) had been doing these things for decades in the US, but we had no idea where to find equipment in South Africa. We started investigating and found out there was a South African father-son team, Team Garwood, who participate in triathlons. Success!

We were so excited to find them because we could learn so much from them and their experiences. I sent a message to them explaining what we wanted to do. Within a few hours, I think, Kevin (Nikki's dad) responded and said they were in Johannesburg and we were more than welcome to come and see what they have when we were close by. It's amazing how things work out, because Mom and I were going to be in Johannesburg for presentations and meetings in a couple of weeks' time. I excitedly replied to Kevin and we made a plan to meet up. We were able to meet their entire family and include them in our journey. They had the buggy at their home, which was awesome. Kevin told us that they were actually looking at new options for Nikki because he had grown too big for the buggy. He said we could take it – we could just organise to courier it to Cape Town. This wasn't the plan, as we were merely going for information and to find out who had made it so that we could get one made for me. It was really special to have them say we could use theirs. We were, and still are, so grateful. They have truly been trailblazers in South Africa, raising awareness and opening minds about what is possible.

When I sat in that buggy, I felt mixed emotions. I was excited because the buggy fit me almost perfectly. (Sometimes being a small human has its perks.) I was also really nervous and stressed because this meant I had one less excuse for not doing the Cycle Tour, as lack of equipment was no longer an issue... We were making progress.

Once the buggy arrived in Cape Town it took a while for us to get on the road with it. We had to extend the rollbar because I was a little taller than Nikki had been when he was using the buggy. (This concerned me. Why would I be rolling anywhere?) We also had to sort out the cushions because I needed extra support to keep me stable in the buggy.

And then of course we needed to name the buggy. We decided it would be "Beastie". This became our team name because Grant is a beast on a bicycle and I am a beast in a buggy. The name now travels with me into whichever sport I take part in. I like it, and it makes me feel badass.
Grant and I started spending time together. If he was going to ride with me and be responsible for helping me with everything I needed on race day, he needed to have an understanding of who I am, what I need and how I think

in everyday life. This turned into a good strategy because he could then determine whether we were in a crisis or not, with minimal communication on my part. He made me feel comfortable wherever we were. I confided in him a lot and we had so many deep conversations about so many things. I remember when we were watching a play, In the Wings, produced by The Chaeli Campaign, and some of the issues explored in the play reflected similar conversations we had had. We sat at the back of the theatre, both of us sobbing.

When Grant fetched me on the morning of our first training ride, I was quiet the whole way to our destination, staring out of the window, looking at the road and thinking about how fast we were going. I was practising the "If I don't voice my stress then it doesn't exist" method – I don't recommend it. After that training ride – we rode over Chapman's Peak and back – Grant realised that that was the first time I had ever done anything at speed. I mean, I've been in cars and stuff, but nothing where I'm out in the open and that close to the ground, with a relatively high level of risk. It was an intense experience for me. It was both stressful and liberating. My inner daredevil was happy.

We worked out some communication strategies to let each other know what was going on. I call Grant "G" because it's easier. Also, just because. We realised that I couldn't always hear him properly from the buggy, so we developed a system of hand gestures and clicking. Our friend Kristina was quite affronted on my behalf that G would click his fingers at me, until we explained the reasons behind it. It was actually a solid strategy because I couldn't see the road ahead of us – Grant was in the way – and it was tough for him to have to yell at me every time there was a pothole or something in the road. So, he clicked at me and pointed in the direction of the thing I needed to be aware of. At least the two of us understood what was happening, even if we confused the hell out of some of the cyclists around us because we used signals that usually don't exist for able-bodied cyclists. Kristina got on board with this signal system after she joined us on a training ride and saw how effective it was. She even started using the click-and-point strategy too. It makes sense.

A few weeks before the Cape Town Cycle Tour I had had my first official ride in Beastie when I took part in Moonlight Mass, which is a night ride through the city, ending at Greenmarket Square. Grant picked me up at my res and asked me how my day had gone as he put me in his car, and I had a complete meltdown. I had just got my first university paper back and I got 0% because when I did my referencing I used full stops instead of commas.

It was time for a good time.

I had been in the buggy before to work out things like the seating, but not while it was attached to a bike and moving, so I was nervous. Moonlight Mass is not that far (a few kilometres), so it was a good introduction to cycling. It also has a rad atmosphere, so I could think less about panicking and just have fun with it. A few things stand out for me from that night. To start with, Grant cycled between two poles and we barely made it through. He was super nonchalant about how stressed I was about riding into stuff, and I was annoyed. He was checking in regularly, so I knew he was still concerned about my wellbeing. I remember staring at a bus next to us, completely silent and just wrapped up in my own thoughts. I was thinking about how I could simply be sucked underneath that bus. It was also quite windy that evening, which made it seem like an even more likely scenario.

When we spoke about it later, Grant mentioned that he had realised how different our perspectives are from the buggy and from the bike. He had a few of these realisations.

One example was when he decided to do a tandem ride and not be the pilot cyclist. He understood, in that moment, the level of trust the person at the back has to have in their pilot, just as I need to in the buggy. Another was the first day of the Double-and-again for Disability – a fundraiser and awareness ride from Hermanus to Cape Town in support of The Chaeli Campaign. It would start in Hermanus on the Friday before the Cape Town Cycle Tour, we'd cycle to Stellenbosch, stay overnight somewhere, and on Saturday we'd cycle from Stellenbosch to the Waterfront. Then on Sunday it was the 109km Cape Town Cycle Tour, which was such a vibe every year. My role had always been to scream at the cyclists as we drove past in the support vehicle. Not this time. This time I was right there in the action. So we were riding and everything was fine, apart from it raining a little, when we spotted a huge baboon chilling on the other side of the road. Naturally, I freaked out. That animal was probably triple my size. Grant's comment to me was, "It's okay, just make yourself big." My reaction? I nearly pooped in my pants. This becomes less of a figure of speech later in this story...

Remember when I said it was raining a little? Well, it went from a pleasant and refreshing drizzle to gross, angry, horizontal storm rain in minutes. It was awful. I was not having a good time at all in the buggy. (Grant wasn't having the best time on his bike either; he always jokes about being a fair-weather cyclist.) After the baboon encounter and the intense rain, my body decided it was time to make a scene. I won't go into all the details, but let's just say we had a situation...

My cycling was over for the day and I spent the rest of the day in the car with Mom, on spectator duty. I was completely drenched from the rain, and once Mom had handled the situation it took forever for me to get warm again. The weather got much worse, and when the cyclists arrived at the hotel where we'd be staying overnight, we welcomed them enthusiastically. Everyone was grateful that the tough day of riding was done and that we could get some proper food into our systems.

[TANGENT]
My friend Juan, his brother Clem and Vilia, their mom (who is also one of our amazing CSRC dancers), joined us for most of the Double-and-again for Disability weekends, to support all the riders. Juan has been a wheelchair user from the age of 19, when he was in a car accident, and has been involved in our work for years. They always brought *gees* or spirit to the support crew mission. I remember a couple of years before this, when Juan and I were lying on the lawn of the place where we were staying, chatting and watching the stars, when we heard rustling in the bushes nearby and we started panicking. Everybody else had gone inside after finishing the braai, leaving us – two disabled people who were unable to move away from anything – to fend for ourselves in the wild. I still don't know what caused the rustling, but we made enough noise to scare whatever it was away and to make a cyclist or two notice that we needed some sort of rescuing.

The 2013 Cape Town Cycle Tour was going to be the first time I would use an indwelling catheter. I was stressed about it because it was new and I wasn't sure what to expect. After an hour or so, when we had settled at the hotel, we decided it was time to put the catheter in and give my body enough time to adjust and get used to having it. Vilia had experience in this area and she offered to help. We were so grateful she was there to help us through that process; she explained everything in detail and made sure I was comfortable. She is a power woman.

[TANGENT OVER]

The next day the weather was stunning and we were thankful. I was especially grateful because I had told Grant how epic the Double-and-again for Disability is, and up to then it had been pretty shitty. It finished strong, though, with a really happy group at the V&A Waterfront. We had lunch with a journalist who was writing about our Cycle Tour because it was the first year that buggy riders were being allowed to participate, after which we went home to nap.

That year, three buggy teams took part. Deirdré Gower had lobbied in previous years to do the race with her son, Damian, in a buggy similar to ours. Her advocacy opened the door to a continued conversation, and now buggy teams are completely accepted and accommodated in the event. The thing about advocacy is that it compounds, and with the determination of a group of people, plans can always be made. Deirdré and Damian are remarkable and have expanded their advocacy with their Warrior on Wheels Foundation, which supports inclusive adventure experiences for disabled people.

So, after working with organisers and having a couple of safety briefings, everybody felt comfortable with and confident about the plan, and we were ready to race.

Grant and I did have a few fights along the way, though. For example, a few weeks before the race Grant and his dad, Gary, were discussing potential exit points. When I joined the discussion (I was feeling left out) and asked why they were talking about this, they told me that we needed to be prepared for every eventuality. I agree that it's important to be prepared. I also believe it's important to take cognisance of where we are focusing our attention while we prepare. To me, planning exit strategies meant they were thinking there was a high likelihood of us failing. For Grant, it was making sure there would be no issues getting help should we ever need it.

This was a huge moment for our friendship and our cycling partnership because we had to acknowledge there are multiple ways to understand or interpret a situation and how important it is to communicate about how we're feeling. We spoke through each of our understandings and reasons, and we found common ground. Ultimately, we agreed that we would only worry about exit strategies if something hectic happened en route to warrant that level of concern and action. We agreed that I understand my body and its limits, and that any decision regarding my body and leaving the race route because of it would include me as a member of the team.

Having a strategy for the possibility that we would have to leave the route prematurely was a good idea. These strategies, we considered, could be devised by the race organisers and were discussed in the safety briefings I mentioned earlier. We agreed that our goal was reaching the finishing line at the end of the 109km route, and we moved forward towards race day with determination to make that a reality.

When race day arrived we were ready to take on the challenge ahead of us. When Grant arrived early that morning with the bike and buggy, he was literally jumping up and down with excitement. My excitement was hiding beneath the fog I felt being awake that early. We got to the start and I had a couple of minutes by myself in the car while G got everything ready. My nerves were all over the place, but I think I held it relatively together. My uncle was there at the start to help some of our hand cyclists with their bikes and later in the day, when we were talking about the race, he commented on how caring Grant is towards me, referencing the way he put sunscreen on my face with so much care...

That day was gorgeous. The weather was perfect and everything worked out the way we wanted. There was so much love and encouragement for our team from spectators, cyclists, officials ... everyone.
We did have one slight catheter crisis on the day. G handled it, though. When I asked him about it later, he said he didn't remember it being that intense, which is funny because that moment is burnt into my mind forever. See? Different perspectives.

We reached the finishing line with just that one drama. Crossing that line was amazing. When we got to the grassy patch the organisers had allocated for us to disembark and change over to my wheelchair we were so excited. A minute later, Grant and I were both in tears. What had we just done? Mom thought G was relieved, but he says that wasn't the reason he got emotional.

We had just achieved an incredible feat, and more than that, the journey leading up to that achievement was made all the more incredible.

G was a game-changer in my life because we met at a time when I was finding my way through feeling that I belonged somewhere after high school; working through how I could and should navigate life with my disability as an adult. It was a time when things could have gone very differently in terms of how I believed I was perceived by others and what I expected of those around me.

He constantly confused me. I wasn't used to people being completely okay with everything relating to my disability. I'd never met someone like this. It was perplexing to me that he had no issues with helping with anything, or taking responsibility for supporting my needs, or making plans to go anywhere, which always has a few more steps than non-disabled plans. All this and more made me question a lot of things I had previously taken as fact. Why was I okay with people not being okay with my disability things? Why was I not expecting more from people? Why was I putting so much pressure on myself to make sure everyone around me wasn't too uncomfortable with my disabled-ness? I hadn't seen or experienced the level of unconditional acceptance that Grant brought. He made me believe it's possible for people to not make disability a barrier; that people can rise to expectations when you're brave enough to have them, because he did.

I had to open my eyes and mind to see that these people exist in more places than I had originally imagined. Once I did this, I found the most unbelievable humans to go on more adventures with me.

Once, when I was on a work trip to Johannesburg, I suddenly felt anxious while we were driving on the N14 and I had a flashback to when we did the 94.7 Cycle Challenge...

[FLASHBACK]
It felt like it was a million degrees Celsius that day. I started and finished that race in tears. The start was Mom's fault (we were super late and she indicated that we probably wouldn't be able to participate) and the finish involved a bit of heatstroke.

Here's the back story:

We had just turned onto the seemingly endless N14 when G took a bathroom break. When he got back, he checked in with me to see whether I was okay, fully expecting me to be. I responded with giggles and questions about the wellbeing of the cows we'd ridden past earlier. I was worried about how they were coping in the hot sun... I was clearly having an adverse reaction to the heat. We had ice packs in the buggy for this purpose.

I was being illogical and arguing with G about everything and he knew he had to do something. After I was cooled down to an acceptable level, we carried on cycling. (We found a balance between G's preparedness and my "it'll be fine" attitude.) The race finish was a few metres after the steepest hill I have ever been on. The heat became too much for me, and the only reaction I had in me was crying. We handled it when we crossed the finishing line and G could get off his bike. He was super calm, but because I was crying, other cyclists had called the medics. It took a few minutes to deal with the heatstroke, but it all worked out. We conquered another challenge and we had more stories to tell, so it was totally worth it.
[FLASHBACK OVER]

After Grant had been riding with me for two years, he got a job in Johannesburg, which meant that he wasn't able to ride with me any more. This was the moment I realised what a big part of my life he had become, how much I trusted him and how much he had opened my eyes to the opportunities and experiences life has to offer, if you're brave enough to embrace them.

For everybody around me, it wasn't even a question. I had to find someone to be my pilot cyclist so that I could keep doing this. Why would I choose not to have these experiences when I had discovered how great they are, and that they are possible? It was harder for me and it was a much bigger crossroads than I realised. I wasn't sure what I wanted. I had to make a decision about whether to continue with cycling or whether it would just be "a thing I did that time". I didn't want to be a hypocrite, but it also felt like a betrayal in a weird kind of way. Like if I just found another person to cycle with me, I would somehow be undermining what we had achieved and the memories we had made, as well as the lessons we had learnt. I didn't know how to close that chapter in my story, and I wasn't sure whether I could cycle with someone else and trust a new person in the way I had trusted Grant.

I lived with this seesaw of ideas for weeks, and eventually I decided that I needed to live some of the lessons that I'd learnt with Grant, one of them being that people will rise to the occasion if you give them the chance to.

Trusting people has been hard for me. This may seem strange because in order to achieve anything in my life, I've had to – to a certain extent – trust other people. But where this becomes tricky for me is that up to that point, not many people had proven that I could trust them, or shown that they would show up if I needed them.

Ed and Brett (also known as Baksteen and Lepel)

Now that I had opened myself and my mind to the possibility that there were many crazy people who would be keen and able to cycle with me, I turned to Facebook and I put out an all-call (this becomes a bit of a trend later) to see if anybody knew anybody. I didn't really expect anyone to respond, maybe because I wasn't fully ready to put my life in somebody else's hands. Sometimes life pushes you and things work out in ways you never expect. Thirty minutes or so after I posted the request, I received a message from Ed.

Ed was originally known to me as "Mr O", as he was my class teacher in Grade 7. I hadn't spoken to him for about five years – since our primary school reunion. It was interesting to call him "Ed" and also to see him in a new light. As a cyclist? I didn't even know that he did the whole cycling thing, but I was excited to see if and how it could work out. We chatted for a while and made a plan to test the buggy with his bike. I was so nervous.

[TANGENT]

After a few weeks of riding with Ed, he told me that he had another idea he'd love me to get involved in and set up a meeting with his friend and colleague, Kevin. Kevin was the head coach for the University of Cape Town's Ikey Tigers rugby team and Ed was an assistant coach. The team had won the league in 2014 in what is arguably the best comeback in the history of the league, and they wanted to include me in their 2015 Varsity Cup campaign.

I thought I'd do a presentation and that would be that. But no. They had bigger plans. I was asked to come through and speak to the team and when

I arrived, we remembered that the venue wasn't accessible from where we had parked. It's a good thing we had a full rugby team with strong, athletic men, and they effortlessly carried me down the narrow stairs in my wheelchair.

I was invited to spend the season on the bench. I got a jersey with the number 24 on it (first supporter off the field). Being a part of this team gave me a sense of belonging that I hadn't expected. I had never taken part in a team sport, so when I was welcomed so warmly I got what everyone was talking about. Even though I wasn't on the field contributing in that way, I felt valued, understood and included. I feel it's fitting with how my life has worked out so far that I found a place to belong in a most unexpected place – in a rugby team. When the boys were playing away games I'd watch from home, but we decided we needed to go and support the team in Bloemfontein for the semi-final. We lost that game, but made some good memories. Many people think I had my priorities wrong because an opportunity came up to advocate at the United Nations in New York, but it coincided with the team's opening game where I was asked to read the Varsity Cup credo. I had already committed to supporting the team and it was important to keep that commitment. I think my priorities were exactly where they needed to be. I have no regrets.

I made some beautiful friendships in that year and we had a lot of fun, especially at the rugby after-parties. Since I was technically an honorary team member, I took part in a few fines meetings, but I physically cannot down a beer (we've tried – it's a mess), so we just exchanged the beer for shots.

Good times.
[TANGENT OVER]

Ed told me that he wanted to bring his friend on board to be a support rider for the Cycle Tour. "The more the merrier," I thought, even though I felt a little anxious. Enter Brett.

The first ride was pretty chilled, I guess. I was nevertheless stressed and I think all of us were a little nervous, but no-one spoke about it. We just needed to take it easy, with no pressure, because it was the first time I was riding with someone else. Also, Brett was sick at the time, so he couldn't be on his bike. He followed us in the car and had FOMO the entire time. He took photos and videos to make sure we had adequate archives of this moment in our history. After a few weeks, when Brett had recovered, we went out on another ride. All together this time.

On this ride everything was going so well and then, as we were heading back to Noordhoek Farm Village for some well-earned coffee and breakfast, it started raining. This was the moment that our new team developed unique nicknames. I think we were trying to distract ourselves from the stark realisation that the weather was hideous and freezing, and my go-to coping mechanism is humour and banter. Ed became "Baksteen" (Afrikaans for "brick") and Brett became "Lepel" (spoon). They call me Poppie. Don't ask me where these nicknames came from. I don't know... Brett is actually usually called "Yster" (which means iron), but for me – and my family – he remains "Lepel".

I think the universe works in beautiful ways and has a way of nudging us towards new experiences. My first Cycle Tour with Baksteen and Lepel was shortened to 47km because of massive fires along the original route. It made it easier for me to move forwards with a mini dose of this new chapter of my cycling adventures.

Lepel became my main cycling partner/pilot and he is a truly special person in my life. He too has been a game-changer. I had never trusted anyone like I had Grant – it took a lot of vulnerability and honesty. My challenge was that I simply tried to transfer how I had worked with G to Lepel. But by doing that I was drawing lots of comparisons, while Lepel worked differently. I had to realise that Grant and I had done something awesome – it was a milestone that opened up my world and made me understand that I was putting my own limitations on what I could do (when there are too many people already doing this). I had to work on myself more to recognise that I had to open my world to allow more people – like Lepel – to bring their own unique magic into my life. Lepel is different and equally exceptional because what he did for me, after the monumental mind shift I'd experienced with G, was to teach me that I can trust other people too; I can rely on other people too. He has helped me to be brave in moving forwards, knowing that each person in my story has a specific place that only they can hold.

I feel like the power of a single person is too often underestimated. I'm not only talking about myself being underestimated, but also how big of an impact a person can have on changing my entire perspective. The best thing is that there are so many opportunities to open our minds and hearts to have significant experiences with people who change our lives for the better.

I've done a few Cape Town Cycle Tours with Lepel now, and when he brought in a new support rider, James, I learnt that we are all far more connected to those around us than we even know.

James and Brett have been friends for a long time and they've taken on different sporting challenges together, so riding with me became a new, exciting challenge for them. I wanted to know more about James and started asking Lepel questions. (I get my interrogation skills from Mom.) I found out that we had been in the same orbit for a while, as James was a teacher at the school I had attended, albeit in the prep school. When I found out his surname, I got excited. As it turns out, James's dad, Tim, was the cameraman the first time The Chaeli Campaign was featured on *Carte Blanche* in 2005. How crazy is that?

IT'S A KIND OF MAGIC

I got into endurance and long-distance running kind of accidentally. I started running in 2015. My first race was a 10km and the running bug bit me and wouldn't let go. I do prefer the longer distances, though. I'm more of an endurance athlete and I feel that doing the longer races makes the logistics more worthwhile for me. I didn't know I would end up loving it as much as I do. I love it because it's a mental challenge as much as it is a physical one. The mental aspect of these challenges is not affected by my physical disability, although some people have told me that the perseverance and resilience I have when it comes to working with my disability every day sets me up well to tackle these endurance events.

Many people believe that when I'm doing physical activities like cycling and running, I'm just chilling in my wheelchair. This is not true. My body is not working as a non-disabled person's would (obviously) and you can't always *see* the work, but it's definitely working. I'm burning energy just sitting upright in my wheelchair on any given day.

Hudson (James)
So, after riding the Cycle Tour with Hudson (oh, I found out that James's first name is actually Hudson, but he generally goes by James, so now I call him Hudson; he calls me Mycroft) he wanted to do another epic adventure. I was relatively open-minded to his suggestions, but when he said we should swim across the Zambezi, I vetoed that one. It was a hard no from me because ... hippos.

[TANGENT]
I've never actually met a hippo, nor do I ever want to, but I've had some near encounters. The first time I nearly met a hippo (I think the likelihood of this happening was far greater in my mind than in reality) was while we were on a camp with our school's environmental club. One of the activities was all about listening to the nature around us. We each had to sit quietly on our own somewhere and pay attention to the sounds we were hearing, and when we came back together as a big group, we'd share our experiences. Simple enough. Then you add the minor detail of my disability, me sitting alone in some tall grass and the comment I had heard a couple of hours earlier: "I wonder when the

hippos are going to come through and say hello." That was a pretty decent recipe for me to set up a panic station, right there in the long grass. This whole activity probably didn't last longer than five minutes, but it was long enough for me to gain a healthy respect for the hippos I'd imagined nearby.

The second (almost) encounter was on a Brownie camp. The camp was really cool and I had a lot of fun that weekend. One night while we were all sleeping in our sleeping bags (this was also the night I woke up to find a frog in my sleeping bag) we were woken up by a loud noise. It was a couple of hippos bumping the jetty outside the camp area. One of the leaders asked me if I wanted to get up to see the hippos. I said no. I'm cool about not having that particular life experience.

[TANGENT OVER]

So Hudson suggested we run the Comrades Marathon (90km between Durban and Pietermaritzburg) and I was keen on that idea. I was looking forward to taking on a new challenge. And it was only a few months away, so we didn't have to wait too long to embark on the adventure. We didn't realise to what extent advocacy would end up being a part of this story...

We entered on the same day we decided we were going to do the race. When we received our entry confirmation emails it seemed like everything was going smoothly. Then I got a message from Hudson asking me if I had read the rules. I had not. Because, you know, that's not the usual order of things. Of course you enter an event you've never done before and then you read the fine print. Obviously.

Confused as to why Hudson had asked me this, I went online to find the rules to the race. And right there, in black and white, it said "No wheelchairs nor mechanical devices allowed". This was a shock to my system because, yes, I'm used to experiencing undercover discrimination and inequality, but here it was so blatant and out in the open for everyone to see. We had entered the 2016 edition of this event and rules like this still existed, and yet we have a Constitution that protects my right not to be discriminated against.

Hudson started speaking about finding other adventure options and very quickly we stopped him from going down that road. This was a big moment.

It was exactly the reason we had to take on this race. We had to fight the discrimination and get them to change the rules. It didn't take too much convincing for Hudson to be 100% on board. After some strategising, we had decided that whatever the Comrades Board decided, we were running. If they said no, we were ready to run unsanctioned. It had been done before – women and people of colour were running unsanctioned for years before the rules were changed to include them in 1975, allowing them to participate equally. So, we knew it was possible.

After weeks of engaging and lobbying, weeks of Comrades saying no and us saying "But yes, because" and a couple of lawyer's letters, we finally got the go-ahead to participate. I think this was a month or so before race day and we had to hustle hard to make sure we had everything we needed to get those Comrades medals around our necks.

This adventure had a different vibe because I wasn't the only wheelchair user involved. Anita – we'd known about each other for a good few years before this – and her legend of a running partner, Hilton, were also invested in making this happen, not just for ourselves as athletes but also for those who will come after us. It's a running joke (pun intended) between us that we are doppelgangers. People confuse us all the time. Not all disabled people look the same, people... That being said, we both have CP and we really do look quite similar. We also have a similar sense of humour.

We wanted to qualify as early in the year as possible so that we met all the entry requirements for Comrades and because I didn't have a proper running wheelchair yet (kind of key to the success of the plan) we wanted to tick off what we could in the meantime.

So I did my qualifying race (we chose Red Hill Marathon in the Western Cape, which happens in January each year) in my mountain-climbing chair. Wheelchairs built for climbing are not built for running. It's like going hiking in high heels. After qualifying in that race, Hilton organised a running chair for me, which was amazing. The plan was that I'd use that chair while training, then Anita would use it for the actual race day and I would have my own one made by then. We know it's not ideal to be swapping equipment like this, but you do what you've got to do. By the time we got the go-ahead from the organisers, we had already asked all the wheelchair manufacturing people if someone could make a running chair for me. Everyone told us there wasn't enough lead time to make one. I must admit I was getting nervous at this point. How would I do the race without a wheelchair? It was non-negotiable – I needed a chair. There had to be someone, somewhere, who could help us. So we expanded our search to people outside of wheelchairs. We found a wonderful man, Zahir, who makes custom-built bikes and other rad wheeled objects through his business, Flying Wheels. He was just crazy enough to agree to make a running chair for me. We found him 12 days before we would be leaving Cape Town to road-trip to Durban. (It was logistically easier to travel by road, with the wheelchairs, but I'm also just a fan of road trips.) He fully believed he could make it happen and I'm so grateful to him for his commitment to our mission of making history. He didn't sleep for too many hours in those 12 days, but he delivered my chair and we were ready for the marathon.

[TANGENT]
You know what they say about new running shoes and marathons? The same rule should apply to wheelchair cushions. We'd been working on the cushions for my running chair for weeks, but we weren't able to test them or wear them in before we left. In hindsight, that was probably a mistake, but we didn't really have an option. So I learnt that hard lesson 25km into the race, when my back started complaining. I think I still have issues from that day, years after the fact.

Now we know.
[TANGENT OVER]

We were given permission to run, but there was a long list of additional conditions or rules laid out by the organisers that only applied to wheelchair athletes. In the final notification emails runners were warned of our presence, as though we were radioactive or something. Many of the rules were said to be for our safety, but it felt more like they were trying to make it as difficult and as complicated as possible to deter future participation.
We are not so easily deterred.

One of the rules was that only one person would be allowed to push my chair for the entire race, and if they found that someone other than the designated runner had pushed me at any point along the route, I would be disqualified (but my runner wouldn't). These rules have changed since then and everything is much more accommodating and welcoming to us as adaptive athletes.

We decided that Hudson would be my designated pilot runner (the runner who would be responsible for pushing my chair the whole time) and Lepel would be our support runner. Support runners, I believe, are crucial team members, not just for bringing more energy to the day but also for helping to get water and anything else the team needs during the race. They are especially helpful in helping to avoid congestion when going through water stations. (This was also listed as one of the organisers' safety concerns.) I feel like non-disabled athletes create more congestion anyway, but that's a discussion for another time. A couple of weeks before race day, Lepel injured himself, but fortunately he was still able to run. Plans were coming together.

We weren't allowed to start in the front (this is now commonplace to ensure the safety of both adaptive and non-disabled athletes), so we started in our respective batches. Anita and Hilton were ahead of us and there were probably 2 000 people between us. It took us eight minutes to cross the starting line simply because there were so many people participating.

Being in the middle of the crowd at that starting line was overwhelming. I feel very tiny in that space. (I mean practically... My perspective is just above people's hips, so being surrounded by thousands of people like that makes me quite claustrophobic.) I therefore have to convince myself that I can in fact still breathe, that it's only intense like that in the beginning and that the crowd will spread out slowly. The music, the energy from all the runners and the realisation of the magnitude of what we were embarking on hit me hard. I was trying to hold back the tears and when I looked back at Hudson and Lepel thinking "Holy shit!" I saw they couldn't hide their emotions either, so I felt better about not keeping it together.

The starting gun goes off and the mass of humanity that I'm now a part of begins to move like a wave. There are a few points in this race where you can take a second to look up and take in the moment. Every so often you can see the thousands of people ahead of you and the thousands of people behind you. It's the quiet moments that get to me. When nobody is speaking and all you can hear are shoes hitting the road. Every person there has their own reasons for taking on this challenge, but it's a collective action, moving forwards one step (or wheel rotation) at a time.

Anita and I had different motivations for doing this race, and over the years we have moved closer to each other's motivation and evolved both of them into a good combination. For Anita, it was about tradition – everyone else in her family had run it and she wanted that experience too. For me, it was about proving to the naysayers that it was possible. Regardless of our individual reasons, when we lined up at that starting line the whole experience was much bigger than just us.

It was about making a point and making it boldly. There were so many people who didn't understand why it was important or didn't think it was possible. We felt the pressure. Throughout the day, we knew the officials and referees were watching us – they would drive past us and slow down, roll down the windows and just look at us (not saying anything, just giving us the once-over), so we felt as though we couldn't give them any reason to say that wheelchair athletes shouldn't participate. We were proving that disabled people are hardcore enough to be there and complete the race. So we made all our own plans – no medical tents for us that year because we didn't want our support needs to be used against us in any way.

There was a lot of confusion and questions from fellow runners. There was also so much support. That's what Comrades is about – helping one another to achieve a shared goal. So many runners said things like "I'm so happy we can share this experience with you" or "It's so awesome to see you on the road; keep going". Not everyone felt the same way, though. We just had to focus on the positive moments. To make positive change, you sometimes have to occupy uncomfortable and hostile environments. I'm used to being in these sorts of spaces. Even though our first year was so hectic, with the level of surveillance and pushback, there is something remarkable about this race that's indescribable; it's transformational.

There's something I call "Comrades Magic", and I'm prepared to bet that anyone reading this who has been a part of this race knows what I'm talking about. Roughly 18 000 people participate every year and I am just one of them. But somehow, people I met at my first Comrades, and didn't see anywhere else, will all of a sudden be next to me on the road in the Comrades. There are people we meet at the Comrades Marathon Expo and chat to for a few minutes, and we jokingly say to them, "See you on the road." What happens? We end up running together – out of thousands of people. What are the odds of that? And it happens year after year. It's magic.

There are too many examples of this kind of magic, but one that stands out for me is this: I had told Hudson and Lepel that anything I had in my running bag had been thought about carefully and was necessary. I'd like to point out that they didn't listen to me and decided to edit what I had put in the bag. There I was, thinking we were completely prepared for any eventuality, when about 2km into the race my front wheel wasn't properly aligned and needed adjusting. I said, "It's all good, there's a spanner in my bag." Wondering why there was no communication coming from either of my partners, I glanced back and they were just looking at each other. "What's wrong, you guys? Just get the spanner." They couldn't get the spanner because in their secret editing process they'd decided we wouldn't need such a thing and had left it in the front footwell of the car. I was so annoyed, but they had created the problem, so they had to figure it out. I was spending my energy elsewhere.

This is where the magic comes in. We had a few conversations about what we were going to do, and needing a spanner. This is simple when you're doing a cycling race because everyone has bike repair kits of some kind. When you're in a running race all people have on them is water bottles, shoes and plasters. We found out that day that broken telephone is an effective and self-starting occurrence at Comrades.

A few kilometres after the first cut-off a couple of runners asked us if we were the ones looking for a spanner. Later on, a few more asked us if we were the people who were looking for someone with a Jeep. What? I was confused. Why did we need someone with a Jeep? The most unbelievable thing happened. Clearly our message had been spread far and wide, and just before we got to our first planned stop, a man called us over, waving a spanner in the air. He was laughing at our confused faces. He told us his friend had called him, explaining that he needed to help us because he has a Jeep. Laughing, he told us that someone on the road had made a joke that if someone has a Jeep, they should also have a spanner. He had both and he was willing to let us keep his spanner in case we needed it later. Apart from that being an amazing expression of Comrades magic, it also made me laugh because that spanner weighed five times as much as the one I had originally packed in the bag.

There was never again any discussion about how much stuff I carry in my bag.

We were so determined to do well and we were ready to turn some heads. We didn't think we would be seeing Anita and Hilton, since they had started ahead of us and are a power team. A few hours in we saw them and then suddenly it was game on! Even though we had a bigger-picture advocacy goal for inclusion of disabled athletes, when we saw each other our competitive sides emerged. People often assume that because we are disabled, we are not competitive. If anything, we're competing every day – with our own bodies, with society, in every environment there is an element of competitiveness – because so many spaces are not inclusive. Anita and I have been competing since we began running. We participate differently from the mainstream, but we definitely have our own personal bests in mind whenever we hit the road and we're definitely always aiming to improve our times. (That's how runners work.)

Throughout the day we passed each other a few times and every time was an exciting point of connection and a reminder of our bigger purpose of the day. It also kept us grounded – a kind of compassionate competitiveness – knowing that the other team was at more or less the same place on the route.

Each year is special and memorable in its own way. I always cry for some reason or other, from happy tears to tears of frustration and pain, and every emotion in between. I didn't think a race could bring out such emotions in me but there I was, on the edge of tears all day.

Two moments stand out for me from that first year.

Remember Lepel had had an injury? It started giving him issues about 55km in, and soon after that he fell behind and we had to make a decision about how we would continue the race. Lepel told us we had to carry on without him because what we were doing was important and he would run at his own pace and find us at the end. I was devastated. Even though he said it was fine I felt terrible about leaving our team member behind. We were meant to finish together, to make history together. I cried for a couple of kilometres and came to terms with the new reality for our team. There is so much support on the road and it really helps us stay motivated, and because wheelchair athletes were a new thing in the Comrades, we had people cheering for us all the way. About 10 or 15km after we had left Lepel, we found our new groove and were working away at the route when we heard someone shout, "Hudson!" We didn't think anything of it because that was the name on Hudson's number, so we just thought it was a spectator showing support. We shouted thank you and carried on. A few paces later, the same voice shouted "Poppie!" There's only one person who calls me that... We looked back and it was Lepel! We got so excited about being reunited that the runners around us also got super pumped, with no idea why, and no idea of the comeback they had just witnessed and been a part of.

It takes time for people to recognise the work I'm doing in my wheelchair when we run. It usually happens after we pass the halfway mark, when fellow runners notice that I'm still engaged and actively participating. My partners have our fellow runners' respect from the start, which is awesome and deserved. It just takes a lot longer for that respect to reach me. It takes a while for people to see me as equally athletic.

For this reason, the next memory stays with me and makes me emotional every time I talk about it. Now reunited as a team, we were about 10km from the finish and we had caught up to the 11-hour bus. (This is a group of runners who run at a certain pace with the aim of finishing in a specified time, so if you don't want to think about your pacing you can just stick with the "bus driver" and they'll get you to the end in time.) We hadn't seen this bus for 10 hours, which blew our minds. When you're on the road for such a long time, you lose track of time and you just focus on moving forwards however you can. When we realised we were behind this bus, we also realised we could come in before said bus, and prove that we are all strong athletes, in our different forms. We decided to go for it and Lepel shouted, "Wheelchair athlete coming through!" It can be pretty difficult to get through these buses when you're stuck behind them, but this time was different. When a few of the runners who were at the back heard and saw us, they moved out of the way and told those ahead of them to do the same. It was a relatively silent action from all of those people, and when we were in the middle of that massive bus, they started applauding us and our efforts. It was a beautiful moment. I felt so appreciated and I felt equal. I was crying and when we had made our way through the bus, Hudson asked me if I was okay. I told him I definitely wasn't and asked him whether he was. He replied, "Not really." That support gave us all the energy we needed to finish strong.

We felt like gladiators coming into the stadium to finish in under 11 hours. The emotions I felt in that moment were akin to the first time I finished the Cape Town Cycle Tour. For about a week, I almost cried every time I thought about what we had achieved.

[TANGENT]
I have not had the same running partners for two years in a row. We all find this pretty funny and often joke that I'm a whole development programme, all by myself. We have counted how many running partners I've had ... and I think we're at 18 so far.

Sure, this could bother me, but it allows me to have so many more epic experiences and share them with more rad people, so that's a win. Sometimes I feel like it would be good to have some consistency and then I realise that I just don't roll like that. I've let go of most of my anxiety around this and I try to focus on embracing the adventure of inviting new, interesting people into these experiences.
[TANGENT OVER]

Ebarnie
In 2017, my second Comrades came around and I thought I was sorted. I had a partner, Paul, and a wheelchair (more than I had had at the same time the year before). I was really excited to try for my Back-to-Back medal for completing two consecutive Comrades Marathons. I am always ready for life to throw metaphorical spanners into my plans. A few months before race day Paul injured himself in the Ironman and couldn't train or run for months, which meant he couldn't run with me.

So again, I turned to Facebook to find some fellow runners. (It was more complicated because we were so close to race day and entries had closed, so whoever ran with me had to have entered and qualified already.) I refused to believe there wasn't one person who would want to run with me.

Two weeks before Comrades I still hadn't secured a pilot runner, but Hilton hustled for me and confirmed an epic pilot runner for my Back-to-Back mission. Ebarnie lives in Bethlehem and was doing Comrades as training for a 100-mile race. Solid choice. I had also confirmed that Sri (who connected with me after he saw my Facebook request) would be our support runner and we'd meet up on the road.

We trained separately and only met the night before the race. We had to work out logistics for the early morning because this was the year Jean Altomari became the first self-propelled wheelchair athlete to complete Comrades (we supported her in advocating for this, as she lives in Philadelphia in the United States and we had already built a working relationship with the organisers) and we had more wheelchairs than usual to manage. I was confident that everything would be fine. I had to trust in Ebarnie's experience.

The next morning we met up at the hotel. We left my motorised wheelchair at the hotel, as we didn't need it at the start since I would go straight into my running chair. Mom went with Jean in the kombi and they had all the chairs – my running chair (it's called Bruce) and Jean's racing chair and everyday chair. I went with Ebarnie and his wife, Daleen, in their car.

Unbeknownst to me, in the early-morning, pre-race chaos we left the cushion for my chair at the hotel. Apparently Mom discovered this when we got to the start and used some colourful language. She dashed back to the hotel to get it. We had learnt our lesson from the first time so we decided to use my everyday gel cushion because my body definitely knew what that one felt like, as it was well and truly tried and tested. I was still sitting in the car, waiting for my wheelchair to be set up, and had no idea what was happening, I just saw Mom rush off. (If you've ever been around at the start of any major race you'll know it's madness and the traffic is next-level.) We had (barely) enough time to sort it out and get to the starting line. We all breathed a sigh of relief when we were in our respective chairs and ready to go.

We always stay at Groundcover in the KwaZulu-Natal Midlands when we do the Comrades (if we're doing the "down" run to Durban we stay there for the duration of the race and if we're doing the "up" run to Pietermaritzburg we stay there after the race) and Mom meets us at the finish. Mom is pretty much always at the end of every race I run. She has what she calls her "dolphin squeal", which seems to be set at a pitch that only I can hear. It's instantly recognisable to me and it cannot be re-created in regular contexts – she only ever reaches this pitch at a finishing line.

I'd planned out my strategy for my bladder and for nutrition, so I felt mostly confident about the day. About two hours into the race I wanted to eat something (I think it was a peanut butter sandwich) and I soon realised that my thoughtfully planned nutrition plan couldn't happen because all my food had been left on the front seat of the car when we did our final check.

I was panicking somewhat and had to have a conversation with myself about my new strategy. I thought, "I've had days where I forgot to eat and it was fine." But those weren't days where I was running 89km for 12 hours. I had to eat and Comrades Magic came through for me once again. Whenever I needed something, someone miraculously happened to come past and offer to share their sustenance with me.

It had been a long day and when we reached the top of Polly Shortts I was so nervous about finishing. We had an hour to do 9km. It was a tall order but Ebarnie is a machine and is so good at pacing, so I had nothing to worry about. We finished the race with eight minutes to spare and I got my Comrades Back-to-Back medal.

What a crazy day. Jean finished in 10 hours or so, which is incredible. She is a phenomenal athlete, with so much grit and determination. She opened a lot of minds that day. People had come round to the idea of wheelchair athletes participating, but Jean broadened the horizon even more, showing the determination and power of disabled people and proving again that there are different ways to perform. Jean is one of the most determined, driven humans I've ever met, and I can't wait to share the road with her again, hopefully soon. I think my best story from that year was listening to fellow runners telling each other about me... Two women were chatting about us while we were walking uphill and I have no idea where they got their information from, but it was entertaining nonetheless. So they said that I was a student at UCT (accurate) and that Ebarnie lived in Bethlehem (still accurate). This is where the story took a wild turn. According to this woman, Ebarnie was my dad (inaccurate and also based on assumptions that disabled people only do things with relatives or significant others...) and because we live in different places, our only opportunity for some father-daughter bonding was to run the Comrades together each year.

I heard her telling this story and looked back at Ebarnie, and all he said was "Ek luister" (Afrikaans for "I'm listening"). It's amazing how people put two and two together and come up with five. I was slightly hysterical. This is why I prefer it when people just ask their questions because otherwise we end up with stories like this one.

A few kilometres from the end we saw a familiar face. It was Muddy Mark. I had met him before because he was dating a friend of mine at the time, so when I saw him, I just said hi and told him to send my love to my friend. After the race I connected with her to find out whether Muddy had made it in time. He had ... with a minute to spare. The stress!

While my friend and I were chatting we decided we should run a marathon together. I don't remember the specifics of what happened, but she ended up not being able to run the planned race with me, so Muddy took her place to run it with me. That was the beginning of a whole new kind of madness – Muddy madness!

Muddy and Stu
My first run with Muddy was the Sanlam Cape Town Marathon and I was planning to use it as a Comrades qualifier, but life decided it was not to be – we missed the cut-off by eight minutes. After the race we were disappointed, but we made another plan – Muddy told me we'd run another marathon later in the year to make sure we qualified for Comrades.

Muddy is a man who goes from zero to a thousand in a minute, and when he commits to something, it's happening. I think this is partly why he was so bleak about our first race. I just saw it as another opportunity to run and make memories; we couldn't change the fact that we hadn't made it in time, so we had to move forwards with new goals. By the time I got home, Muddy had messaged me to say he could run the Winelands Marathon in Stellenbosch with me. Within five minutes of getting that message I got another one saying he was keen to run the Comrades with me the following year. That level and speed of commitment was new to me, but it's become something that I really appreciate. Muddy is always ready to go on an adventure and change perceptions. Interestingly, people have assumed he is my dad on a few occasions. (Sometimes I call him Pops, just for fun.)

When it was time for the Winelands Marathon, Muddy told me he had invited his friend, Stu, to be a support runner, and confirmed that he was also a beast of a human. I hadn't met Stu yet, but we would meet on the road. He wasn't allowed to start with us, so he just had to catch up. It only took him about 5km to get to us and our introduction to each other was memorable, at least for me.

As usual, I had an indwelling catheter for the marathon. Mom put it in the night before because it takes a while and we had to be up pretty early. It wasn't the best catheter moment – sometimes the body just isn't as on board as it should be. I was uncomfortable from the minute I woke up. We were constantly adjusting the pipes and so on to get the correct position right up until I left with Muddy to head to the start. We waved to Stu in the traffic as we went and he and Muddy shared some hand signals I didn't understand, and we were on our way. By the time we reached the start, Muddy had already readjusted my catheter once, under the light of a streetlamp.

We started the race with the usual two-minute head start to avoid congestion at the start. The officials sent us the wrong way (this happens a lot more often than people think), so Stu had less work to do to catch up. A few minutes after we had started running, I knew there was still something strange happening with my catheter. It just wasn't comfortable and when it's correctly placed there shouldn't be any pressure in my bladder and definitely no urge to wee. I had both. So while we were getting kilometres in the bag I was silently trying to figure out what the issue could be. We'd already repositioned the pipes, so in my mind it couldn't be that. I thought we should take a little pressure off my bladder by removing some of the water in the balloon. (This balloon sits at the end of the catheter inside my bladder and, when filled, it stops the catheter from falling out – important!) There's always a lot of give and take when we're on the road, and we were coming up for the 5km mark, so Muddy and I agreed we'd sort the balloon out when we reached that mark.

We saw the 5km board and crossed the road to a safe space to solve my problem. Muddy was focused and went into problem-solving mode, getting all the required supplies from my bag, and it was at this moment that Stu caught up with us. I officially met Stu while Muddy had his hands in my pants holding a syringe. Perfect. Welcome to disability, Stu. I don't know what he thought was happening, but we didn't talk about it. Whenever I have stopped in a race people get very concerned (and I appreciate the concern) and ask whether we need anything or if they can help in any way. Everything was fine, we just needed to adjust things once again. So without many words between us, Stu took on the role of telling everyone that everything was fine and there was nothing to worry about... "Nothing to see here, folks."

Muddy removed a small amount of water from the balloon and it felt better because there was less pressure. I felt like we'd solved the problem. But 10 minutes later I realised this was not the case.

Long story short, I spent most of the race trying to come up with possible reasons for the catheter problem. Eventually I decided that the catheter was blocked and it would eventually leak and overflow, and we could deal with the mess later. Just after the halfway mark I couldn't deal with the pressure any more (I was cramping, ugly sweating, crying and still slightly mortified that this was my introduction to Stu) and I decided that the only solution was to take out the catheter. I obviously didn't want to take my pants off on the side of a road in Stellenbosch, but we'd devised a strategy that didn't require such action. But as Muddy was loosening the strap on the leg bag to remove the catheter, ta-da! Instant relief. What was happening? Turns out there was nothing wrong with the catheter itself, it was simply a kink in the bag that had blocked the flow. Such a simple solution. I cried out of frustration and annoyance. Ridiculous.

The rest of the race was rather uneventful and we finished a few minutes inside the cut-off time. We all exhaled deeply, excited that we had achieved our goal for the day despite a small Chaeli Crisis.

At this point in my life I feel like one of my love languages is coping with a crisis...

Anyway, we had now qualified for Comrades and could commence with some serious training. Our training strategy was simply to enter all the marathons and longish races to figure out what we were doing, in a marathon setting. That worked for us. We just didn't realise how close together the marathons were scheduled. It was a little intense, but that's on brand, so it's all good. People began recognising us as a team and that was awesome. This was a big deal for me because up to that moment my running journey had been all over the show, with different pilot and support runners. Don't get me wrong, I have loved running with each of my running partners. There's something powerful, though, about having specific people consistently show up for you and with you. Muddy and Stu have always understood the bigger picture of the advocacy embedded in my running mission, and they've always been ready to fight those battles with me. I know each of them would never let anything bad happen to me while they're around. I know I'm safe and that kind of security is not always easy to find.

[TANGENT]
In one of the races we did (not a marathon) there was a referee who rode so close to us on his motorbike all morning that he nearly knocked my wheelchair. Muddy and Stu both shared some strong words with him, but he was relatively unfazed.

Both of these men have beautiful hearts. Muddy has a bit of a short fuse (just don't be shitty and ignorant at 5am at a starting line), but I still see Muddy as a sort of chocolate Caramello Bear – hard exterior but soft on the inside. Stu is a little different. He is super calm and will go with the flow, but don't push him. And then there's me. So, this referee dude was working on our collective last nerve.

About 5km from the end the referee was back on our case and asked for Stu's number. When we asked why, he told us that Stu was going to be disqualified because he was running "outside the lines". Have you ever tried to run with a wheelchair on a pavement, avoiding streetlamps and thousands of other runners? So yes, we were running outside the lines, but it was the safest option for everyone – for us and our fellow runners. When I objected and pointed out that I too (the wheelchair athlete who is the reason for us nudging the rules) was running outside the lines and should therefore also be disqualified, suddenly this referee was far less interested in the whole disqualification thing. And that, my friends, is an example of ableism.

[TANGENT OVER]

Muddy suffered a hamstring injury at the Two Oceans Marathon, but was still committed to running Comrades (remember the Muddy mantra, commit and make it happen). Given this development, we decided Stu would be the pilot runner. For the past two years it had been the rule that only one person could push me for the entire race, so we were planning and strategising accordingly. We had continued the dialogue with the organisers and each year the rules are reconfirmed and sent out in the final race info pack. This rule had now changed, which meant that Muddy would be allowed to assist and share the responsibility of pilot runner. Progress.

I feel like this particular year's Comrades was the hardest one yet for me – physically, mentally and emotionally.

When we started early in the morning we were running in complete darkness and when the batches came through I remember feeling anxious that somebody was going to run into my wheels and trip and injure themselves. It was stressful because it was so dark that I couldn't even see my front wheel. It was an intense hour or so. When the sun came up I think I exhaled properly for the first time.

The morning of the race was cold, but it was set to warm up to comfortable not too long after the sun came up. So I wore minimal layers for the morning – I figured that adrenaline would keep me warm until the sun could. I was wrong about this. I am not great at regulating my body temperature and because it didn't get warm or sunny until midday, I was freezing. I kept trying to embrace the mind over matter mantra and "think warm thoughts". It didn't work at all. The cold had made its way into my bones and I knew it was there to stay. I noticed how hectic it was when I asked for a peanut butter sandwich and struggled to lift it to put it in my mouth. I felt like rigor mortis was setting in. Clearly that was my mind being overdramatic, but movement was difficult in that moment (more so than usual).

I usually have it together throughout the Comrades, with the odd session of tears. I was already crying at 23km and I was humbled many times that day. I didn't want to be that person who couldn't deal with life this early in an ultramarathon because if you're struggling at that point, you know it's going to be a rough day. By now, through all the training and races, Muddy and Stu know me pretty well. I was feeling really sensitive and when Stu asked me, "Chaels, are you struggling?" I realised that I actually was, but I didn't say anything. Muddy saw my eyes welling up, looked at me, put his hand on my shoulder and said, "My girl, you're fine," and a couple of minutes later, "Remember, you have three minutes." Important reminder. I nodded while the tears rolled down my face. I knew I was fine, but it didn't feel like it at the time. I managed to pull myself towards myself and after a while I felt as though I was defrosting.

I think my brain went into "cold mode" and didn't register when I was physically overheating; my body was hot (I was working, after all), but in my mind I was still freezing. So for the first half I was freezing and for the rest of the time I was nauseous. I didn't understand why that was happening, so we stopped to check in. It was warmer now, so Stu unzipped my jacket, thinking that maybe I was getting hot. It was like I had turned into a sauna! My body was so temperature-confused and was trying to tell me there was a problem by making me nauseous, but I wasn't paying attention to the signals. At first I thought it was a bladder thing, so I asked Stu to check my catheter bag. That was when we discovered my catheter hadn't been closed properly and it was flowing all the way; I was leaving a trail along the route – like we were leaving breadcrumbs for Muddy. Ha ha! It had also been running into my shoe for the two hours since we last emptied the bag. It reminded me of how embarrassed I had been the first time Hudson had emptied my bag onto the road, but this time I wasn't embarrassed at all, I was in ultramarathon survival mode. We could sort out my shoe later. Now, we just needed to get to the end.

It never crossed my mind to call it a day. We just needed to keep moving forwards and to keep counting down the kilometres. I was miserable, but we were moving. We had mini goals that were marked by where Stacey, Stu's fiancée, was supporting along the route. We started bargaining with ourselves: "If we get to this place in the race, then we can have..."), and our next goal was getting to Stacey at 62km. I was so happy to see her when we got there. I was mostly happy to keep still so my nausea could stabilise. While Stu sourced a sandwich from a spectator, I leant my head back against my headrest, just breathing, with my arms stretched out on my wheels. I think Stacey was slightly unsure of how to support me just then, and when Stu got back she told him I needed help. I really appreciate this next moment...

He just asked me what I needed. I took a breath and said, "I need to vomit." Everyone else around us was quite concerned, but Stu told me that was cool and manoeuvred me and my chair backwards onto a piece of grass and said something like, "You've got two minutes." I can neither confirm nor deny that I threw up on said grassy patch, but we waited for my anti-nausea meds to kick in and then we were on our way again. Those worked for approximately seven minutes. Stu offered me some chicken mayo sandwich but I wanted nothing to do with mayonnaise at that stage.

I always feel like the last 5km are the longest in races and it was definitely the case here. When Stu phoned Stacey to give a status update we found out that Muddy's hamstring had been giving him too many problems and he had decided that if he continued, he'd be creating a long-term injury, so he would meet us at the finish.

I was so emotional at the end. Coming into the stadium is always emotional, but this time I felt physically ill, and the fact that a member of our team was waiting for us in the stands tore at my heart. When we crossed the finishing line (with about 15 minutes in the bag), I was feeling so nauseous that I thought I was going to pass out. Based on my previous experience I thought we would finish, get our medals and get out with minimal attention, but it wasn't like that at all. To our complete surprise, there were cameras, interviewers and even flowers for us. That was so amazing and unexpected, and I'm so happy that we've reached this stage of acceptance and celebration at Comrades. It's so much bigger than just being allowed to enter and participate in the race. Comrades is known as "The Ultimate Human Race", and so what they've done is to recognise our humanity as disabled people and adaptive athletes.

We experienced the full spectrum of emotions during the day's events, with so much wonderful banter. And when we met up with Muddy, it was the most emotional reunion ever. I was crying, he was crying, Mom was definitely crying. And it was beautiful. It's one of my most vivid memories from that day.

I have had special experiences with these two men and I am so grateful. It is always a total party whenever they are around and they are always making crazy plans for more adventures. Anything is possible when you refuse to believe that it isn't. That's exactly how they work, and when they are making these plans that energy is compounded and I can't help but get excited too. Apart from the adventures, I have shared some of the deepest, most meaningful conversations with both of them. They make space for my thoughts to run away from me and then help me to rein those thoughts back in.

[TANGENT]
Muddy and I had intended to spend a weekend climbing mountains in Cape Town, but things happened and we had to postpone it, and then life happened and it was delayed for the better half of a year. We made a plan, Mud came down from Joburg for the weekend, and we were going to do Lion's Head and Table Mountain via Platteklip Gorge. (We'd already climbed Devil's Peak, so we wanted to do the other two big peaks in Cape Town together.)

This ended up being the same weekend that Damian passed away. It was so good for me to have something planned for the day after his death because I process grief and loss by doing things... What better place to be when trying to appreciate life and its beauty than on the side of a magnificent mountain? When Muddy lost his footing a little, my initial response was one of anxiety, but in trying to get a handle on that, my mind spiralled into the massive loss we'd experienced the night before. Mountains, for me, are places of peace, reflection and power, where you can feel whatever you're feeling. I was processing my pain, and it manifested in a complete breakdown while I was on Muddy's back, with many concerned climbers witnessing it. Mud just sat down on a rock and gave me that moment. I don't know if he fully knew how much I appreciate that day. It was a hard day on many levels, but I left that mountain with an immense sense of peace. When I'm feeling overwhelmed, I often find myself thinking back to that day.
[TANGENT OVER]

Once we were back at the car in the parking lot after the Comrades, we could finally start talking about all the crazy and beautiful things that had happened during the day. We met our fellow CSRC runner, Earl, on the road at about 30km, in the middle of my crises and deep into my running wall. (My wall starts at 26km and lasts for about 3km, during which time I can't and don't talk to anyone.) I'll admit that I wasn't the best version of myself just then.

Earl ran the Two Oceans Marathon in 2018 with a charity entry, raising funds for Inclusive Arts Collective. After that he became a member of the CSRC Running Club and did his first Comrades that same year as a CSRC runner. He ran a 10km race with one of our wonderful Chaeli Campaign beneficiaries, Kudzai, and he was hooked. Earl loves being part of these moments and is always ready to help wherever he can. I don't think he knew what he was getting into when he offered to run my next Comrades with me, though!

Earl and Chantal
After a few conversations about Earl being a pilot runner, off I went on a new adventure with him. Chantal, also a runner, then came on board as our support runner.

We've grown a lot as a team, as well as when it comes to understanding one another. Everybody has a story and a journey. Running is something that connects people and offers opportunities of reflection, humility and triumph. On one of our training runs, Earl told me that starting running saved his life. It's such a powerful force for finding new aspects of yourself and for personal growth, and often challenges you to achieve things you didn't think possible and to grow in ways you weren't expecting.

When Chantal joined the team, her catch phrase was "I'm scared". I loved that she was so open about her uncertainty. Open communication is one of the most important things in an adaptive athlete's team. Now, after being my pilot runner a few times, she is a complete boss on the road. I speak a lot about finding your voice (both metaphorically and physically) through doing all this active stuff, and that applies to all of us. I had to find my voice – and use it – to make sure people knew I was there. I remember the day we did a half-marathon and Chantal found her voice and used it properly and forcefully! It was incredible to be there to witness that moment. I looked back at her and thought, "People better get out of this woman's way." Powerful.

We decided to do the Sanlam Cape Town Marathon in September to qualify for the 2019 Comrades. Chantal and Earl came to pick me up at our house and then we all went together because I can't handle the anxiety of not knowing where my partners are at the start of a marathon. My wheels were a little flat, so we stopped at a petrol station before heading to the start. We arrived at our predetermined parking spot and when my jogger (this is what we call the running chairs, so please don't call them prams – we're adults) was put together, we noticed that the left back wheel was flatter than it was after we had pumped it up at the petrol station. Now, I'm not blaming Earl for this dilemma... All I'm saying is that he was the only person to leave the vehicle and the only person to touch the wheels during the time in question. (Don't worry, we've spoken through this and we're all clear and happy about what happened.) Either way, no air was staying in this tyre. We didn't have time to figure this out because we were now running late, so we figured we would find solutions as we went.

We met Anita and Hilton at the start and told them about our problem. We were still pretty confident we would find a solution in the not too distant future. We quickly discovered how difficult it is to run with one flat tyre. There was a garage along the route, so we thought that might be our saving grace, but alas, the valve was too far gone, so we had to devise a new plan. That plan involved Mom bringing a different set of wheels from another jogger because Earl still had those wheels in his car from a race he'd done with Kudzai. (Luckily Earl had left his keys with Mom.) We ran a half-marathon distance with the flat tyre because it was the closest point Mom could get to. After solving the tyre problem, we thought we were good to go, but apparently not. We turned the corner after our quick pit stop to get the new wheels and ran straight into a headwind. A few difficult kilometres followed, and Earl mentioned how sticky the brakes were. We had just had them completely redone, so we just put it down to a rough day with a stubborn wheelchair. If anything, we have learnt that every piece of equipment has a personality and attitude of its own, and it deserves (and demands) respect. When Chantal took over from Earl, it was still a struggle and we figured the chair wasn't agreeing with the weather and was making our lives difficult. As it turned out, none of those assumptions was accurate. The headwind coincided with a downhill, so Earl had put the brakes on and when the road levelled out, he forgot about it and we ran for 7km with the brakes on. After a couple of minutes of Earl being in the dog box, we were all laughing about it.

Our 2019 Two Oceans Marathon experience was, quite frankly, a disaster from start to finish. We arrived too early (and I'm not being sarcastic when I say this was very unlike us) and it was raining, although admittedly not heavily. I didn't want to stay in the front seat of the car for the whole time, so Earl put me in the boot of the kombi and we all sat and waited for the time to pass. I was sitting very comfortably when I suddenly spasmed, lost my balance and tried to stop myself from falling over, but my hand slipped off the edge of the boot and I nearly fell on my head. The only reason I didn't fall out of the car was because my jogger was in the way. Nobody noticed until I made more of a scene that involved some screaming and slight swearing. So that was a great start...

We were given a five-minute head start and I think about 15m into the race something happened with my front wheel. It was making a strange noise, so Earl checked it out and attempted to fix the problem. He underestimated his strength and when he adjusted the wheel the central pin snapped. This is the part that keeps the front wheel attached to the rest of the chair, so it's kind of important. We freaked out. We had barely started, and it felt as though our race was already over, or at least significantly jeopardised. Nobody was answering their phones and we realised _we_ had to find a solution. We made our way to a nearby garage to see if they had anything we could use to "MacGyver" my wheelchair back together. They had cable ties (it was so early in the morning that it was miraculous that it was even open and that there were people there) and a number of spectators came over to assist us. One man who helped us had done a couple of Ironman events and we could see he had definitely put his bike together with things that don't generally keep bikes together. We appreciated his knowledge and experience so much. The way everything was attached meant that the flag we use to bring more attention to our existence could no longer be placed where it usually would. Whoever was the support runner would just have to carry it.

By the time my wheel was sufficiently attached (not terribly securely, but it was there) 20 minutes had gone by and our head start meant nothing. When we got moving again the officials had already started opening the roads and we were literally the last people in the race. We didn't think we were going to finish or even see another runner for the rest of that day. When we eventually found a fellow runner, we were so shocked that we were instantly re-energised and motivated to get going. We were actually still in the race!

We felt pretty good for most of the race after that stressful start. When we reached the top of Ou Kaapse Weg my brakes very conveniently stopped working. It's a pretty steep downhill road with lots of bends and sharp turns. To say we were panicking is an understatement. We must have been sending out "please help us" vibes because even though we hadn't verbalised anything, the ambulance was behind us, escorting us to level ground. It's as though they knew chaos was potentially imminent.

We finished the race within the cut-off time and we felt we had achieved the impossible.

When we went to do Comrades in 2019, we all agreed that Earl was not going to adjust anything on the wheelchair. We all felt this was the best strategy for success. For the whole road trip from Cape Town we were so excited – making plans and strategising. It was Earl's attempt at a Back-to-Back medal, Chantal's first Comrades and my fourth. So, there was pressure on multiple levels, but we were prepared to take on the challenge.

We got to the start and there was a buzz. It's always a beautiful mixture of excitement, panic, silent hesitation and loud determination. We'd decided that Chantal would be pushing me at the start, which I thought was so epic. It was a true reflection of women power and I was all for that!

The previous day we had met a man at the Comrades Marathon Expo. He sat down at the same table as us and we started chatting. He and Chantal connected over their shared nervousness; it was his first Comrades too. When we left, I said we'd see him on the road, and he laughed. He didn't believe me – he didn't know about the magic yet. Never underestimate the magic! Early in the race, we were chatting among ourselves as a team and we heard someone say with a laugh, "Ag, no man." We turned and saw the man we had seen the day before. He looked at us in shock, and all I said was, "I told you, it's magic," and we laughed and hugged. It was awesome.

We had made it through the first few cut-off points and every time we did we exhaled, celebrated and checked our strategy. We were going with a strategy of picking up the pace for the second half of the race. It would have worked, but we were slightly off with our timing. We misjudged the terrain around the halfway cut-off. Going into halfway is a downhill, and downhills are not necessarily faster with a wheelchair, because much more control is needed, so you can end up going slower than you think you will. We could see the board saying we'd made it halfway. We heard the cut-off gun and reached the halfway mark (42km) 90 seconds too late.

We were devastated. None of us was making eye contact or speaking with anyone. The realisation came in waves. We heard people pleading with officials to let us keep going. People were crying, swearing ... any and all reactions were happening around us. I guess what we experienced there was equality. There are no exceptions – if you're too late, you're too late. That's fine. I can appreciate it, but it still hurts.

It is a special type of sadness that's saved for these moments. Each of us in the team felt responsible for not making it. The guilt and disappointment ran deep into the soul. Apart from the team being completely broken, it felt like the stakes were higher for us, considering the battle we'd had up to that point to be accepted in the race, and the fact that we were representing wheelchair athletes and were still proving ourselves. We failed in our mission (that day) and I finally understood how Anita felt two years earlier when she and Hilton missed a cut-off.

I had to get out of the herd of sadness, so Earl pushed me onto the grass and left me on my own for a bit to process what was happening, while he had a cigarette. I don't know where Chantal was, but wherever she was, she was sobbing. I hadn't started crying yet. I was just thinking, going over everything I did that took up time. Thoughts like "If I hadn't asked to take off my jacket, we would've made it" flashed through my mind. Later, when we could use words without breaking down in tears, I discovered that Chantal and Earl were having the same thoughts about their own actions.

While I was sitting on my own one of the officials came over to me and I think she could feel my heartache. She hugged me and said, "We're still so proud of you." That was it, I was done – I had joined Chantal in the sobbing station. So, we all came back together and cried (and swore just a little) together. I'm pretty sure there's footage somewhere.

While we were in the middle of our Team Beastie breakdown, a plan was being hatched to get us back home. We were of no help and weren't really keen to help anyway because this was not *our* plan. We weren't even tired and sore; we still had another marathon in us.

The race officials stationed at that point organised a separate sweep vehicle because we couldn't go in the bus with everyone else, as my chair wouldn't fit in the bus. I think the process that followed was more traumatic than not making it in time and being forced to finish our race early. Before you're allowed to go anywhere, an official comes to you and notes down your number so they can record that you didn't make it past that point. Then, before you get into the bus or any vehicle, like in our case, a different official comes to you with a pair of scissors and they cut your number in half, off your chest. I get it – they have to make sure that no one sneaks back into the race – but what a way to twist the knife!

After my number was cut off me, Earl put me in the sweep vehicle and my chair still didn't fit, so they had to dismantle it. I was a crying mess and it felt like each piece of my wheelchair that was removed and placed on the seat behind me was a piece of me. That sounds dramatic now as I write this, but at the time it really felt like they were dismantling my Comrades dreams.

The final bit of emotional turmoil was that for some reason we weren't able to use back roads, so the only way to get to the end was to follow the route. We had to finish the race in a car, with my chair in pieces on the seat behind me. Even though it was painful, we could see all these wonderful people making it happen. We were so happy for them but still so bleak for ourselves.

After sleeping on it, we were back to planning for next time. Earl made the point that we had a DNF, which means Did Not Finish, but he said we could redefine it; we could change what it means to us. We could change it to "Do Not Forget" instead. It did take us a minute – and a drink (or two) – to get to this point of acceptance, but we got there.

When we arrived home, still disappointed that we hadn't achieved what we had set out to, Dad came out with his quiet pride and some solid "Dad advice" and perspective. He told me that having this happen gives me more credibility and legitimacy as an athlete because we didn't make it. That didn't make sense to me initially, and then he explained his thoughts more... It proves that it's not just luck, it's work. Every athlete has races or events that don't go their way or according to plan, and we're no different. A wheelchair doesn't change that. And as long as you learnt something it's worthwhile, even if you don't have a medal to show for it.

This was a hard lesson to learn, but sometimes these kinds of lessons are the ones that shape us the most. Sometimes, when we don't get what we want or the world says something isn't for us, it gives us more resolve and fire than achieving it ever could.

We are so determined to go back and dance over that halfway mark cut-off and prove that we can come back strong and fierce. It's uncertain when that will be because no races are happening yet owing to the Covid-19 pandemic, but we're ready. And when it's safe to do so, we will be right there on the starting line singing the national anthem, getting goose bumps when *Chariots of Fire* plays and crying with joy and gratitude that we can once again have the privilege of sharing the magic with strangers who become Comrades.

Going for green

Usually people want to "go for gold", but when you're a runner it's all about going for green! When you've successfully completed 10 Comrades you get a Green Number or permanent number. (This system applies to other marathon events too.) I've decided I need to get my Green Number for Comrades. This is a personal goal, and it's important for advocacy and for solidifying the place of adaptive, assisted athletes in the race. When you have a Green Number, your name goes on a wall at the Comrades Marathon Expo, so nobody would be able to deny our presence or pretend that it wasn't that big of a deal.

We're here and we're not going anywhere.

Finding Freedom through Fitness

As I have mentioned before, I have always worked with my body through therapies and disability-related activities. When Muddy and Stu convinced me to give CrossFit a go, I was nervous and anxious. There would be new people, expecting new things of me, and I didn't actually know what to expect. I had done some internet searches to see how CrossFit works when you are disabled, but I didn't see people with my level of disability. I saw non-disabled people competing at the CrossFit Games (these are like the Olympics for CrossFit), lifting their body weight, and then some... I was pretty terrified. That's not me, and it gave me more anxiety about trying CrossFit. I found out just how wrong my perception was. Yes, those people do exist in the CrossFit community, but they definitely don't make up the majority. Everybody who walks (or is carried, like me) into the gym has their own fitness journey and that's the baseline standard that you work with. This was a whole different mindset for me: focusing on functional fitness, where my disability is a factor (not a reason for doing the activity) that can always be accommodated and workouts can always be adapted to my level of ability. This is an attitude that's not readily practised in everyday life. It shows me, though, that it is possible – now all we have to do is translate this attitude into every space in society. Simple, right? Not so much, but we can work towards it every day.

I didn't know how much CrossFit would change my life and my relationship with my body and my disability. We organised a session with Marco (a coach and biokineticist) at The Bloc, a fitness facility in Cape Town, and it was the best decision ever.

The first thing that happened when I arrived was that I was taken out of my wheelchair and put on the floor. Marco wanted to see what we were working with. In my online research I'd only seen people doing things in their wheelchairs, so this move took me by surprise. My wheelchair is my safe space, my area of control, and now I didn't have that. I felt vulnerable. I have never appreciated being on the floor (remember my worries of falling over as a toddler from the first chapter?); I've never understood why people elect to sit on the floor instead of grabbing a chair from nearby. I'm still not 100% sure, but I'm closer to appreciating it than I was before. It's not as limiting as I thought. In the context of my fitness it is enabling because I have many more options for moving.

It took me a while to learn this and feel comfortable enough on the floor to get my body to do what we were asking of it.

That first session will stay in my mind forever, especially now, years later, considering that the work we did then is now a warm-up for me – that's when I realise the growth and achievements.

Marco wanted to get a baseline of my ability, to see what we were working with, and I was surprised how difficult it was to do the exercises. I think this is also why I wasn't a huge fan of floor work. It made me feel super disabled. He asked me to roll over, from my back to my side and back again. Then we would see how many of those I could do. It took me eight minutes to do one. It was exhausting and frustrating. We have this moment on video. I felt as though I was never going to get to the other side...

I think we all realised then how much more effort it is to get my body to cooperate and do what I want it to do. I had to learn how to channel my frustrations around my body's lack of interest in working with me into something constructive.

[TANGENT]
On a positive note, I started these CrossFit sessions towards the end of the year, so when we were all on holiday I could work on doing these fundamentals and go back the following year having gained some more efficiency in all of these skills. I worked on the moves virtually every day for three weeks – rolling from side to side and lying on my tummy to get my hips to calm down and relax. (I was pretty much a right angle.)
[TANGENT OVER]

When it comes to my body and my brain learning new things, it's all about repetition – finding the movement process and then doing that over and over again so that it sticks. For many of the things I do in CrossFit, my neural pathways don't exist, so we're building the connections slowly but surely.

In the beginning, I was anxious because I felt like I had to explain how my body works. (This is no different to any other day or place.) Muddy was there for the first few sessions, which made me feel more chilled because he knew me. This made me feel less pressure to be on top of it, because I actually had no idea what I was doing. There have been many times in my life when I've had to trust strangers, and here was another space where that was needed. Obviously, Marco isn't a stranger any more, and we've figured out how to communicate and get the best out of my body (when it's feeling cooperative and when it's not).

One of the first things I learnt in CrossFit is how to fall safely without injuring myself too badly. I am very effective at the falling thing. I do it constantly. I'm not great at protective reflexes like putting my hands up in front of me when I inevitably fall over, but I'm getting better at it. This challenge of literally finding my balance has been more a psychological challenge for me. If I'm feeling uncertain or nervous about what I'm trying to do, it's hard to focus on not falling, making it all the more likely that I will fall. Sometimes I have to work hard to concentrate on what I'm wanting my body to do, instead of focusing all my attention on not falling.

Sometimes learning something new is a group effort, for example when we were working on me moving from lying down to sitting up. Sounds simple enough, doesn't it? I don't know exactly how many muscles you use to sit up from a lying position, but I do know it's a whole lot of them. I needed to figure out how to make all those muscles do what I wanted, in the required sequence (coordination is tricky with CP), to enable me to do that movement. When I was staring blankly at Marco, I think he realised that this was a moment for more show than tell. So there he was, with Muddy too, lying alongside me on the floor attempting to isolate each step – and possible alternative steps – in order to find a strategy that might work for me. We have since learnt that the best way for me to figure it out is to work it out within my own body, but I have to admit that watching the two of them rolling around in slow motion like a pair of sloths will be endlessly entertaining to me. I also feel it's a great reminder that when things are not working as planned, take a break, go back to the basics and do one thing at a time.

Movement is far more complicated and complex than many realise because for many people it comes naturally and they don't have challenges with moving. When things are simple and don't require much thought, people tend not to see the effort it could be for others.

Now, years later, I ask things like, "Which muscles am I talking to for this one?" I can then get to working on my uncooperative neural pathways.

Whenever I'm sorting these messages from my brain to my muscles, I'm sure the people around me can see there's an inner dialogue taking place. I appreciate that they just let me have that conversation with myself and not try to offer suggestions in that moment. When my strategies are not working for me, I'm totally ready for input, but I like to give it a go myself first.

Every time I go to the box we work on something new, mostly because my body decides on the day whether the strategy we created the week before is the right one for that particular day. It isn't always. I've learnt so much about my body; how it works and how it can work. The small successes and changes are just as valuable and celebrated as the big ones. I feel like I can be successful in this space because it's a supportive environment where I'm encouraged to embrace my doubts and the fear that I'm going to fall on my face and break my cheekbone or give myself a concussion from falling and hitting my head on one of the uprights. (This has not happened as yet, but there's still time…) I'm learning to trust that my body will learn and that deep down, it knows what it's doing. Patience is hard when my mind knows what to do but my body asks, "What do you mean?"

Marco's mantra is to work with the body you have today. I have taken this on board and have to remind myself of this on those hard days.

I use the lessons from my experiences working with other disabled people, for example the wheelchair dancers at the CSRC.

Marco often just waits in our sessions, watching me work (I guess this *is* his job), giving me time to converse with my body and come up with a plan to get the work done. I appreciate him making space for this process because it gives me an opportunity to have autonomy over my body, even if it takes a minute. Too often, disabled people are told, through other people's actions and responses ("It's okay, I'll just do it for you, don't worry"), that we take too long to get things done. I don't have that here. If I'm getting annoyed with how long I'm taking to do a new movement, Marco's right there with the reassurance that if that's the only thing we do that day, it's perfectly acceptable. You know you are having a good session and are on track when you hear Marco say, "That's power."

Together with CrossFit, I started going to Body20, a company that focuses on electrical muscle stimulation (EMS) training. I think this is a powerful fitness combination that is working for me. The targeted electrical impulses (these are not painful) help to activate the desired muscles to do particular movements. Because of my CP, my muscles activate randomly (spasms), so this helps me to coordinate my brain and my muscles. It's also helpful for circulation, which can be problematic in my life, so that's awesome. I remember doing EMS a few times when I was little to see what the baseline of my muscle responsiveness was, and it was really interesting to get information about my body function at that level. What I do now with Body20 is to work consistently to remind my muscles how they can (and often do) work.

I have learnt that life is a whole lot of trial and error, and that each of us has a unique makeup, and we have to find the systems, strategies and combinations that work for our particular design. I believe that being active is a mindset, and we can make choices every day to be active – whatever that looks like to you.

The key message I hope people take away from my fitness journey is to have more faith in your body. It's going to be with you for your whole life, so it's a good relationship to work on.

It's not just about sharing the wins; it's important to share the hard times too. Sharing the shitty moments where I'm questioning everything and feeling super frustrated has been the best way for me to find the people who can support me to overcome all those self-limiting beliefs that sneak into my headspace. You don't have to be a completely open book, telling every person you meet all of your business. You get to decide what you share and what you keep private. Even if you don't have complete control over what people need to help you with, like me, it's still possible to have a say in how you are helped and how you exist in the spaces you occupy.
I have found that finding my fitness has led me to a space of freedom. I feel empowered that I have the power to control my body (even though it takes a while sometimes). I feel free to explore and push the boundaries of my previously expected limitations. I've found a sense of community not only at the box but also online, where I'm sharing the process of finding more function through fitness. The people who have been following since the beginning have been a part of the journey – from feeling hopeless and not

being able to get my body to work with me, to feeling like I have a proper handle on doing my workouts to the best of my ability and seeing that work translate into everyday activities like picking up a bottle off a table becoming easier, or staying stable in the front seat of a car without panicking.

People can relate to the challenges and struggles and so many have reached out to me to connect, sharing their stories too. The struggles are part of the story and make the successes all the sweeter.

Majestic Mount Kilimanjaro – *pole pole*

Never underestimate the power of a little banter at a braai...

I never thought that a seemingly unimportant and random conversation in 2011 would lead to one of the most unbelievably meaningful experiences of my life, with me becoming the first female quadriplegic to summit Mount Kilimanjaro. It did take four years to get there. (We finally made it to the mountain in 2015.) Climbing a majestic mountain like Kilimanjaro is such a privilege and I realised just how great a privilege it was the moment we got out of the bus at the foot of the mountain. You can feel her power instantly.

There are too many stories within stories about my Kilimanjaro adventure for me to share them all here, as they would take up a whole book on their own. (Watch this space!) But I'm going to let you in on just a few of the big lessons and some of my memories from this epic adventure.

Teamwork makes the dream work
The first lesson of this adventure is to know when people are being serious and when they're talking about doing something without actually intending to do it. When we were throwing around ideas of things that would be cool to do in a lifetime, I didn't take the conversation too seriously – climbing Kilimanjaro was just a cool idea.

Over the four years the team ebbed and flowed. It only started taking its true shape about a year before we were scheduled to climb. People got excited about it when I told them about the plan, but life happens and many couldn't take part in the end. It's all good – I also got stressed when it became more than just an idea. This happened when Adam (he lives in the same neighbourhood as we do but he was essentially a stranger at this point) contacted The Chaeli Campaign because he wanted to climb Kilimanjaro and do it for a cause. He came for a coffee at our headquarters and chatted to Mom. When she was conducting her friendly interrogation, she found out that Adam lives about five minutes from our home, and would see us leaving in the mornings when he was taking his children to school. Mom told Adam that I had been talking and thinking about climbing Kili too. And just like that, we were seriously climbing this mountain.

When we decided that we were indeed going to embark on this adventure that we weren't 100% sure how to tackle, our team started to grow. We put out a call to our networks to find people who'd be keen to join the journey. We ended up with a team of nine people, including a cameraman from SABC's *Fokus*, Danie Hefers, to document this historic moment. Danie joined three days before we left Cape Town. The group was made up of people with diverse life experiences and that made for so much more learning and growth. Everyone had amazing stories to share and lessons to teach. There was never a dull moment on the mountain, as most of us didn't know one another, so every story was new and interesting. It also meant that each of us, being so different, responded uniquely to the challenges on the mountain.

Everyone has a role in achieving a goal. Kilimanjaro taught us that this role can totally change depending on the situation. We can't be tied to any ideas of how people are going to engage because anything can change at any minute. We have to be flexible and adaptable, both as a team and as individuals.

My intended role was to bring positivity in the tough moments. Finding the positive in something is usually a skill I'm great at. We didn't realise that emotions flow and fluctuate differently on a mountain compared with in everyday life. There was not a single moment when we were all feeling the same, so everyone needed positivity at different times and at different levels. With this newly acquired knowledge we realised that even though we were supporting one another to reach our goals for the climb, we couldn't be rigid about who was doing what. I couldn't be the positive one for everyone – we all needed to share the responsibility for maintaining team morale. Everyone stepped into the space they needed to when they needed to, and that made us a stronger team in the end.

The best-case scenario for us would have been for everyone in the team to reach Uhuru Peak. However, we knew there was a strong possibility that this wouldn't happen, given the statistics on how many people make it to the top. We were determined for as many of us to summit as possible, especially because we felt that our mission with the climb was bigger than us summiting, it was about shutting down the haters and the naysayers, and proving that things are possible. Two team members were sent down the mountain for different health reasons – Anne on day four and Johanna when we reached base camp. Each time a team member left the mountain we were really sad and it became extra motivation for us to keep going. The biggest lesson here is that each person has their own mountains to climb (metaphorically and physically), and not everyone's mountain includes a summit. It's all about the journey and the lessons learnt along the way.

Trust and communication on this trip were a whirlwind of learning and figuring out how to do things together in the most efficient way possible. I've spoken about how important this is for me in previous chapters and this was a challenge when climbing Kili.

Whenever we talk about climbing Kilimanjaro, an inevitable question Mom gets is, "Did you go up with her?" The answer is no. Mom doesn't want to climb mountains. She did arrive in Tanzania a few days after us, to facilitate inclusion workshops at Village of Hope Mwanza, and it was nice to know she was nearby. We had met Julius Kenyamanyara, the director at Village of Hope Mwanza, a year or so earlier, and he had invited Mom to run empowerment workshops with them. She had an amazing time and we've continued our relationship with Village of Hope through The Chaeli Campaign's Therapies programme.

On our flight to Joburg (the first leg of the trip) I realised how intense this thing was. I'm not even talking about the massive mountain right now. I was travelling to a different country with people I basically didn't know, apart from Taylor, who was studying with me; we'd been friends for about a year. Pretty risky when I think back on it, but I guess it was another calculated risk. And everything worked out fine. I'd told everyone to be prepared for some wheelchair drama (based on almost every previous travel story) and they said I was being overdramatic. That was until we got to Nairobi, when Adam and Taylor watched the ground staff frantically attempting to put a wheel back on the wheelchair after it had fallen off the luggage carousel. Fortunately the wheelchair arrived in one piece in Tanzania.

When we arrived in Tanzania we also discovered that Carel, our team leader, who had been family friends with Taylor's family forever, and Sally, Carel's partner and fellow badass adventurer, had had some difficulty explaining why they were travelling with a wheelchair when they clearly didn't need one. Carel and Sally had left a couple of days before the rest of the team to sort out all the logistics. We had decided it was smart for them to take Scotty (that's the name of my mountain climbing chair) in case there was an issue and we needed time to fix anything on Scotty before we started climbing. On our arrival, Taylor also had to help me explain to the customs person in Swahili that it wasn't possible for me to stand up for the identity photo. It basically took a while for all of us to get on the same page...

It's amazing how much you can learn and grow when you don't have any other options. The moment I hugged my friends and family goodbye at the airport and we walked through security, we were on this adventure and whatever happened, we would have to make a plan. And although we had had many conversations about what my needs were, theoretically, it's a completely different thing when you have to put theoretical strategies into practice. This was the first time I was solely responsible for effectively communicating my needs. In every other adventure I'd embarked on, there had always been someone who knew me nearby in case of a serious crisis, but not this time. I don't think that was as daunting to me when we reached the mountain as it was during the journey to the mountain. There was a lot of time to run through worst-case scenarios in my mind (bad idea – I don't recommend this) and I didn't share those with my team. As a result, I internalised my anxiety for about a day while we were travelling, but once we landed at Kilimanjaro International Airport that went away and my mindset shifted to "Let's do this!"

I was reminded a few times by various team members that I have to use my words, I can't just make a noise and expect people to know what I'm asking for. (That came later.) After a couple of days we'd all worked out a communication strategy that was functional for us and this in particular was a huge moment of empowerment for me that I've taken into other aspects of my life.

Just breathe
When you're climbing a mountain like Kilimanjaro, many would assume that that is the only thing you are thinking about; that the goal is the only thing on your mind.

I didn't experience it that way.

That mountain is a lot to take in and she asks a lot of you. It's constantly overwhelming. It's important to pay attention to what's happening around you, and it's equally important to pay attention to what's happening within yourself – how you're feeling, what you're thinking – and sharing this with your team members. We learnt more about one another than anyone was ready for. Having this attitude in our team led to a sense of connectedness that was crucial for enabling us to make it through the climb. We had to be present for one another to keep us all safe, and we had to have one another's back.

I'm used to relying on others to support me through life and I'm used to things taking longer. Everything *anyone* does when you're on a mountain requires much more energy and takes five times longer than usual. Each movement requires a deep breath – and breathing was harder, especially when we got to the higher altitudes. Seeing everyone struggling with everyday tasks like tying their shoelaces or pulling on their pants gave us all a new perspective.

I'm not sure if I had the advantage. I deal with my body's lack of cooperation on a daily basis, so in a way maybe I was more prepared for that part than the others. At the same time, I need more energy than non-disabled people to do things even when I'm at sea level, so it could also have been no advantage at all. Either way, we learnt that it's okay just to sit with it and breathe in the moment. Getting frustrated is fine, but we still need to move forwards.

I realised while we were climbing Kilimanjaro that I really do like breathing. I had never understood this before I found myself on this mountain, consciously having to take a breath. I grew a new appreciation for my body and the things that it *does* do without me thinking about it. It got harder to breathe as we went higher, and taking those conscious breaths and being purposeful about it became a good grounding exercise, keeping me present and focused on what we were there to do.

A few times I did think I might die on the mountain. (I know this might sound a little dramatic, but it's how I felt!) The worst thing to do is to panic – I forgot this in those moments – and then to forget to breathe.

The first time I thought there was a possibility I might die was on my 21st birthday...
[TANGENT]
Yes, I turned 21 on Kilimanjaro. It was an epic way to celebrate that milestone birthday! I was so happy to be there and wake up to that incredible mountain, and all the guides and porters made it such a special day. There was a lot of singing, which was beautiful, and they even made a cake on the mountain. It was definitely a birthday to remember.

We hadn't planned this as a birthday excursion. Not at all. We planned the trip for that week because it coincided with our university holidays and so that we wouldn't miss any classes or need to request any concessions. (Look at us being responsible students – ha ha ha!) Two weeks after we got back I had a party to celebrate not just my birthday but also our Kilimanjaro climb. We had a really good time. In all honesty, I think we may have had too much of a good time, considering the hangover I had the next day. We temporarily forgot that we – "we" being me and my Kili team, who all came to the party, which meant a lot to me – were probably the fittest we'd ever been from climbing a giant mountain and had unintentionally become lightweights. (At least, that was what happened to me.)
[TANGENT OVER]

There was a bit of miscommunication between me and the guides who were carrying me, and I ended up parallel to the ground on top of a giant boulder. Carel had to practise some tough love just then, because I was freaking out and hyperventilating. I calmed down after a couple of minutes of being right-side up on solid ground.
The day we made it to base camp was a pretty intense one. To start with, on the way to base camp I didn't notice that some snow had got into my shoe and was freezing my foot. Because I don't have great temperature regulation, it was quite a thing to warm up at base camp, but we managed to make it happen. I had a delayed reaction to all of this, only panicking about it when everything had been handled and sorted. I had a complete panic attack in my tent while we were meant to be "resting and preparing to climb". My brain simply said, "Nope, we're not doing that!" so Thembi, who is a super businesswoman and was my tent buddy, had her work cut out for her that day because my body was being

completely otherwise. She helped calm me down and reminded me to breathe.

A couple of hours before we were going to prepare to leave for the summit, my catheter blocked. (Fortunately, I knew this was the problem because it's happened before.) Usually we would take it out and put in a new one, but that wasn't possible for various reasons, so we flushed it multiple times and that seemed to do the trick. I was so frustrated and annoyed with my body for deciding to do this at the last minute. There were so many other moments it could have chosen, but I guess it could also have been so much worse. It could have blocked while we were climbing in the pitch-black, minus-degree weather.

The last hectic thing that went down before we left for the summit was Johanna getting really sick and being sent down the mountain. She had decided, because of a few factors, that she would stay at base camp and not attempt the summit. The plan was that she'd stay there, wait for us and then come down with the whole team. But her body had other plans. There are lots of logistics to figure out when someone gets sent down, but the team leaders were great at keeping everyone calm. When Johanna got down she was examined at the hospital and given the all-clear. She arrived at the hotel a couple of days before the rest of the team. Mom was already waiting there for the team, so she and Johanna were able to share stories and welcome us all back to the hotel, where we all shared a well-earned cry and Kilimanjaro beer!

I had told Thembi about my intended mantra for keeping me focused while we were summiting. Many years before, I'd watched the movie *Why I Wore Lipstick to my Mastectomy*, which is based on the memoir of the same name by Geralyn Lucas, who was diagnosed with breast cancer in her twenties. In the movie they shared Geralyn's mantra for when she was struggling, and it's really stuck with me. I didn't plan this ahead of time, but it felt apt to use in the moment. I couldn't remember the full quote on the mountain, but I got the gist of it. Here's the full quote:

I am the sky and nothing can stick to me. The sky is open and vast and stays unchanged no matter what; it is always the sky. A storm can roll through it, an airplane can roar through, and it is always the sky.

When you keep telling yourself "I am the sky" and you look up and see nothing but pitch blackness, it can be tricky to navigate the emotions that come up, but this was still so powerful for me. It reminded me of our bigger purpose with the climb, especially when it became really unpleasant and difficult.

We had been climbing for what felt like hours. It was completely dark and it was getting colder and colder. Every move forwards was celebrated (internally) and we were one step closer to the top. We had found a good rhythm of rotating guides to avoid exhaustion and make sure that we kept motivation as high as possible. (It was more of a quiet resolve at this point because there was no spare energy for excitement.) Every step required immense effort and the terrain was especially difficult because it was scree and it moved underfoot, so where you stepped wasn't actually where you stayed – you always ended up a bit further back. Anyway, so we were making our way one scree step at a time and Ola, who was the guide in charge of the team that was working specifically with me, slipped on the scree and skidded what was probably only a few metres backwards. As a safety precaution, we had attached my wheelchair to the guides in case Scotty slipped. We hadn't thought about what would happen if one of the guides slipped...

It felt as though we were falling down the mountain. The guides got a grip on Scotty and we stabilised. A good number of choice words left my mouth in the pitch blackness in the early hours of that morning. It was a really stressful moment, and we didn't speak about it that much afterwards. We only told my family about it months after we got back home when Taylor brought it up at a braai. We chose not to share certain parts of our climb... When we got down from the mountain and I had a chance to speak to my family, the first thing I said was, "Look, I didn't die!" Little did they know we had survived some pretty hairy moments.

Leave it as you found it, and leave forever changed
Kilimanjaro demands respect. She is not there to be conquered, she is there to be appreciated and to be regarded with awe. I don't think I fully grasped this in the beginning, but it didn't take long. If you don't approach Kili with this kind of attitude, I don't believe you can be successful. Kili will put you in your place and show you her power; you'll learn a hard life lesson. I know this sounds very philosophical. It is the

journey that this mountain took me on and I'm so grateful for all the lessons I learnt there. It is not possible to experience this majestic mountain and not to change in some way. For me it was a truly transformational time of my life. It may have only been a week, but it was a week that forced me to grow like I have never grown before.

We did a combination route, designed in a way that made the most sense for climbing with a wheelchair. We also had an extra day for acclimatising. It was very helpful to have a day to "relax" – not that this is truly possible on a mountain like Kilimanjaro, but still. It also gave us the opportunity to take some time to do something special for my family. We made a family decision that it was a great place and time to spread my Gran's ashes. (She had passed away some years before and we hadn't found the right way to do this.) She was able to be with me on my 21st – something she had spoken about wanting – and she got to go on an amazing adventure with me.

The route was remarkable. If you speak to anyone who has climbed Kili, they will tell you how every day is different and about how the terrain changes as you go higher up. We started out in lush forests with little monkeys watching us from the treetops, then found ourselves on grey rocky paths, with amazing (and some terrifying) bugs that I've never seen anywhere else. Each phase is beautiful in its own way and it felt like we were walking through a story – one that we were also adding to – and each new kind of terrain was like a new chapter to explore and uncover. None of these was easy with my wheelchair, they were all just varying levels of difficult. The guides we had were phenomenal and without their commitment we would not have been able to achieve our goal of reaching the top of Africa. Guides and porters really are the unsung heroes of climbing expeditions.

Mountains, I've learnt, are sacred places. They stand steadfast and offer us a place for deep reflection and contemplation that can't be found anywhere else. So much of the time you spend on the mountain is quiet time, where everyone around you is moving forwards, quietly and *pole pole* (slowly, slowly). There is a connectedness to your team and to the mountain, but also with yourself in a powerful way. If you want to figure out who you are, go and find a mountain – she'll share some insights. Mountains take you along a path of thinking about your life, your choices, your priorities, everything. When we woke up, got out of our tents and found ourselves sitting between two sets of clouds, I gained so much perspective. It was one of the most transformational moments in my life and I don't think I have ever felt such a sense of peace as I did that morning. Big "aha" moments don't always come with fireworks and fan clubs – they're often sneaky and silent. It doesn't have to be loud to be profound.

Perspective comes with Kili whether you're ready or not. We were spending so much time with ourselves and our thoughts (it got pretty intense for me in those dark times, when we had to dig deep to find motivation to keep going), and as we worked through those thoughts we were learning about ourselves. We learnt about what we thought our limits were and we surpassed them. Every time I got to a point where I felt it was too much, I took a much-needed deep breath and moved past that self-doubt. Even though I overwhelmingly and fundamentally believe that I am capable of achieving whatever I put my mind to, I still have doubt dragons following me around that I have to fight off every so often.

I'm so grateful for my Kilimanjaro experience. It allowed me to prove to myself that I'm so much more capable, stronger and braver than I thought I was.

When we left base camp at 11.18pm to head towards Uhuru Peak, it was the start of the longest, hardest day of my life. I have never felt so many emotions at the same time, good and bad, and I wouldn't change it for anything.

Many people know about me because I climbed Kili in a wheelchair. If that was the reason for you picking up this book, I love that. I apologise if you were expecting more details and stories about the nitty-gritty stuff of this adventure. I'll share those next time. For me, some of the biggest lessons I've ever learnt took place while we were climbing Kilimanjaro and experiencing all the associated trials, struggles and triumphs.

I've been on numerous adventures so far and I'm sure there will be many more in my future. One thing I know for sure is that bringing people with you on your life journey is much more fun than going it alone. Yes, I am powerful in my own right and it's a daily commitment to remind myself of this, but when I forget this or I am struggling, I can lean on the people around me. They are remarkable, special human beings who help me to do amazing things and I cherish them for adding so much to my life. It's a powerful feeling knowing that while I cannot control everything, I, in all my disabled glory, can share my vulnerabilities with others. In this way I can be my whole self, wherever I find myself.

Unapologetically,

Chaeli
X X

Made in the USA
Columbia, SC
30 September 2021

46052254R00137